THE

Keep It.
HEALTHY

PROSTATE

PLAYBOOK

A/PROF CRAIG ALLINGHAM
MEN'S HEALTH & SPORTS PHYSIOTHERAPIST

THE PROSTATE PLAYBOOK
Published by Redsok International
PO Box 1881, Buderim, Qld. Australia. 4556

3rd Floor, 14 Hanover Street, Mayfair, London, UK W1S 1YH

2019
www.redsok.com

NATIONAL
LIBRARY
OF AUSTRALIA

A catalogue record for this
book is available from the
National Library of Australia

ISBN: 978-0-9870766-7-0

Disclaimer
This book is not a substitute for examination or treatment by a qualified health professional. This book contains information of a general nature and does not purport to be an evidence based medical text. Following any advice or recommendations is no guarantee of freedom from prostate cancer or associated complications. The publisher, author and distributors expressly disclaim any liability to any person for any injury, inconvenience or complication sustained, or for any use or misuse of any information contained in this book. The author has made every effort to provide accurate and clear information in the book, and cannot be responsible for any misinformation. This disclaimer extends to any linked or third party content referred to in this text.
This book is a work of non-fiction. The author asserts his moral rights.

Images on pages 13, 15, 16, 20, 31, 32, 41, 42, 57, 60, 65 sourced and acknowledged from Wikimedia Commons.

Acknowledgments
The author is extremely grateful for the time and expertise of those who helped in the preparation of this book:
Mary O'Dwyer, Maggie Allingham, Peb Blackwell, Dr Michael Gillman, Peter Dornan AM, Joanne Milios, Tina & George Clyne.
Cover Design: 99 Designs

CONTENTS

KEEP IT. HEALTHY

Every man has a prostate gland and wants to keep it. And the best way to keep it is to ensure it remains healthy.

A diagnosis of prostate cancer confirms that your prostate gland is far from healthy and may require attention from a surgeon, oncologist, radiotherapy or other curative program. Or you may be diagnosed with a low-risk, slow growing prostate cancer for which Active Surveillance may be the treatment of choice.

Two main problems with prostate cancer are the possibility of it metastasizing (seeding cancers in more vital organs) and the side effects of interventional treatments which can include incontinence, loss of erectile function, depression, extreme fatigue, mood changes and body temperature surges. All of which reduce quality of life.

As a man with an increased genetic risk of prostate cancer I am keen to reduce all the risk factors within my control, to make the gland a cancer-hostile environment. This Playbook is my strategic plan for success and I share it in the hope that you, me and our sons will not fall victim to cancer in an organ that is not vital and should not be a cause of death.

When prostate cancer is prevented or contained there is no urgent need for removal, radiation or chemical castration. It remains in place while you live around it. In fact, it might just be the kick you need to make life-prolonging changes across your health choices.

THE PROSTATE PLAYBOOK is your strategic guide to avoid treatment for prostate cancer. Even if you have it.

Asst. Prof. Craig Allingham APAM
B.App.Sci(Physio), Grad.Dip.Sports Sci., Cert.Men's Hlth, Exec.MBA
Men's Health & Sports Physiotherapist

WHY A PLAYBOOK?

When I joined Australian Baseball as National Team Physiotherapist I was asked to contribute to the team playbook. 'What's a playbook?', I asked, and learned it was the instruction manual for success. The team playbook contains strategic and tactical information for all team members, such as training drills, positional skills, in-game tactics and communication signals.

My contribution included injury prevention strategies, strength and fitness programs, performance nutrition and hydration guidelines, travel skills, injury management, supplement and medication guidelines to comply with doping rules and other resources to help all the players be at their best on game day.

The Prostate Playbook has the same goal - to prepare you for game day. And every day is game day as you prepare for a long season of game days.

This is a play-by-play instruction manual to improve your understanding of your prostate gland and how you can keep it. Healthy. This playbook has the strategies and tactics for you to manage prostate cancer to minimise the chance of progression or spread. Or to protect against getting the disease in the first place if you are at risk or just want to be prepared.

You are in a training program for your life. Your success will be determined by your mindset, your persistence, your learning and application of skills, your moment-to-moment decision making, your support team and your masculine stubbornness about staying alive to do stuff.

THE PROSTATE PLAYBOOK will help you outwit, outplay and out-survive prostate cancer. But you have to turn up and play the game.

USING THIS PLAYBOOK

Read it

All of it. Start at the beginning, stop when it does your head in, then come back and read the rest. Even when you read things you don't like, don't agree with or think don't apply to you. Read other stuff as well. Listen to your medical team and family. Talk to your mates. Then read this playbook again, it may not include all the answers, but it will help you navigate your prostate cancer journey no matter how the game twists and turns.

Know yourself

Review your skills. Have you the determination, persistence, support, confidence, knowledge and stubborness needed to give this your best shot? If not, this program may not be for you. A half-hearted effort will ensure half-arsed results. If it all sounds too difficult or you think you might start next week, you will probably fail.

Turn Up

Not just on the easy days. Stick with the program on the difficult, embarrassing and inconvenient days. Alter priorities, create time in your schedule, change habits and preferences even though nothing appears to be changing, because when nothing is changing, you are winning.

Be Open

Be coachable and open to new options. Keep your filter open and you will learn valuable information. Everything in your life so far has led to where you are now. If you have cancer, it is a clear message to change something. Unbelievable as it sounds, you may not know everything yet. I sure don't.

There is no Championship Game

The Prostate Playbook is for life. Your life. There is no end-of-season championship game and no off-season where you can take a break from the program.

Regular monitoring

If you are already diagnosed with prostate disease, or acknowledged to be at risk, it is your responsibility to monitor any changes in your prostate status. Your medical team will indicate which tests may need to be done and how often. Their goal is to identify when to switch to active treatment. Your goal is to confound them at every turn by staying well and keeping your prostate as healthy as possible.

> *You can train your body to be cancer-friendly or cancer-hostile.*
>
> *One path is easy, the other is a daily challenge to be the best man you can be for as long as possible.*

Offensive Strategies

Through this book are actions or activities that you will need to start executing. These are the offensive strategies in the playbook and might include taking up a type of exercise or including a new food in your diet.

Defensive Strategies

There are also the activities or habits you need to cease or reduce which make up your defensive strategies in the playbook. These might include foods or drinks you eliminate from your diet or reducing your work stress.

Your ultimate success will rely on both Offensive and Defensive adjustments to your current plays. It is important that you have strategies from both sides. as there is no point kicking goals if you keep conceding them.

Not succeeding does not mean you failed

No playbook will guarantee success. No team or athlete wins every game or event he enters. Sometimes the opposition gets the upper hand and even the best strategies come up short.

If you are on Active Surveillance (page 15) you may experience pressure to start treatment for your prostate cancer instead of just accepting it and working on your health. This pressure may come from medical professionals, your family or your own worries about which is the right path for you. Eventually the diagnostic test scores from the surveillance may leave you no alternative than to undergo treatment.

This is not a failure on your part. Prostate cancer is an unpredictable and frustrating disease. Some men will stay on Active Surveillance (AS) for the rest of their lives, some will have to move on to surgery, radiotherapy, chemotherapy, androgen deprivation therapy or some new therapy still in development. Not because they have failed, but because their situation changed. Despite following this playbook and implementing their best possible game plan, the opponent got ahead.

The time and energy you invest in this Playbook program will repay you whatever your subsequent pathway. If treatment becomes necessary, you will arrive in much better health with reserve capacity in your immune system, mental strength and preparedness knowing you have done all that was possible to avoid it.

Just as importantly, you will undergo treatment for the cancer having already learned and implemented powerful physical, dietary and mental strategies that will continue to repay your commitment what ever treatment you undergo. Not only might it improve your post-treatment outcome, but will also boost your defence against heart disease, stroke, cognitive decline, diabetes and a host of other diseases.

If your treatment appears successful in removing or radiating the gland there is still a possibility of recurrence if any prostate cancer cells have escaped beyond the gland prior to or during treatment. These Playbook strategies may reduce your risk of developing aggressive and life threatening secondary tumours elsewhere in your body. No guarantees, but it certainly won't increase your risk.

THE PROSTATE GLAND

Anatomy and Function

The prostate gland is about the size of an average walnut (around 35ml) and is wrapped in a network of fibrous tissue invested with blood vessels and erectile nerves on their way to the penis. The gland is located directly below the bladder, sharing a muscular connection where the urethra exits the bladder and passes through the prostate gland.

The prostate gland produces semen, the milky-white fluid that provides nutrition for your sperm cells. This is added to fluid from the seminal vesicles which makes up the transport medium for the sperm. The final mix emerging from the prostate into the urethra provides both the environment and the nutrition for sperm cells after ejaculation.

During ejaculation, the prostate acts as a muscular pump to provide the sperm with an assisted start to make their journey easier. A valve in the prostatic urethra below the bladder ensures that urine flow is blocked during ejaculation.

Manufactured in the testicles, the sperm are matured in the epididymis of the testes where the acidic environment keeps them inactive. From

Male Reproductive System

pubic bone
ductus deferens
penis
urethra

seminal vesicle
bladder
prostate gland

epididymis
testis
scrotum

there they move through the ductus (vas) deferens tubes to the seminal vesicles.

The role of the prostate is life-generating but not life-essential. It plays no vital part in keeping you alive, which is why it can be removed surgically with no need for supplements or implants.

This doesn't mean removal of a prostate gland is undertaken lightly. It is a complex surgery which can damage nearby nerves and blood vessels and the prostate connection with the bladder and urethra. It is true that technology (e.g. robotic surgery), diagnostic accuracy (MRI) and surgical skills for prostate removal are constantly improving, yet it remains a technically difficult procedure. Challenging enough for surgeons to usually leave the prostate in place during the already complex male-to-female transgender surgery.

A cancer that stays in the prostate will not be your cause of death. Well not directly. It won't compromise any vital function you need for survival, however it might worry you (stress), distract your immune system and leave you vulnerable to other conditions or simply be an advance message that your current health strategies are not working and other problems are just around the corner.

Life without a prostate gland or living with a prostate tumour does not compromise your masculinity. Your sperm production and testosterone levels are independent of its activity unless you undergo androgen deprivation therapy (ADT).

Finally a word about **Prostate Specific Antigen** (PSA). This is a natural substance produced by the prostate gland as part of semen and is necessary to release the travelling sperm from their gel (semenogelin) enabling them to pursue the target egg.

Tiny amounts of PSA leak into the blood stream from prostate cells and can be detected in your blood test. Low levels are considered normal but sustained higher PSA levels indicate the prostate gland is either irritated due to infection (prostatitis), getting larger or growing a cancer. Temporary rises in PSA can occur after ejaculation (the prostate pump squeezes PSA into the blood flow), physical massage or compression of the gland. Re-testing under different conditions usually shows a return to baseline levels of PSA for a normal prostate.

CANCER

Understanding the Opponent

What is cancer? Where did it come from? Why you? These questions are often unasked as you try to absorb the news that you actually have prostate cancer. Your immediate concerns relate to diagnostic numbers, treatment options and the impact on your life, relationships, finances and work.

Understanding cancer may help you deal with these concerns by adding knowledge to your emotional response. Arming yourself with an understanding of the opponent will enable you to identify opportunities to undermine its strengths when selecting strategies and tactics.

Rebuild and Renew

Every minute of every day we are replacing cells in our body that have reached their use-by date. This happens throughout the body - skin cells, brain cells, artery cells, kidney cells, bone cells and prostate cells.

Replacement cells are produced by splitting a cell of the same type. This process involves 'unzipping' the DNA genetic coding that defines the structure and function of that cell, and putting each half of this unzipping into a budding cell nucleus where it is promptly reconstructed into a full version of the original DNA. This process is remarkably accurate, producing a new, healthy cell fully programmed to get its job done.

The 're-zipped' DNA in the new cell provides the architectural blueprint to complete the rebuilding of the cell. All the bio-machinery of the cell is constructed including the energy production system, the storage organelles and the waste removal system. Each cell also has its functional aspects, DNA directs a muscle cell to construct contractile proteins so it can shorten, bone cells are told to build calcium frameworks, gut lining cells to build transfer systems to bring dissolved foodstuff across the cell membranes and your brain cells are directed to build connections to nearby cells to pass messages.

The cell rebuilding process is resource dependent: it requires raw materials in the form of proteins, fats, carbohydrates, minerals and vitamins that you deliver through what you choose to eat or drink. The better quality your daily nutrition, the better quality are the micro-ingredients delivered for cell building. If what you eat has indadequate or poor quality nutrition, you are rebuilding with poor quality materials. Your new cells may be less resilient from the get go.

This DNA division and rebuild happens millions of times per day in your body across all your cell types and occasionally there is an error when the DNA copy is not exactly like the previous version. This is a mutation - a new cell with a less than perfect DNA replication.

Faulty DNA means the cell is different, its genetic code is wrong and it can't do its job. In fact, it may not even be able to keep itself alive and promptly dies. This happens daily throughout your body and the dead cell is broken up by other cells (doing their job) and any useful elements recycled elsewhere. The mutated DNA is destroyed.

Cancer cells occur at random in our body, including the prostate, and most of these cells die because their DNA is either incompatible with life or they become victims of a 'search and destroy' mission from our immune system defence which recognises the DNA error as foreign.

But some survive. Occasionally the mutated DNA in a new cell is not fatal in its own right, nor is it so different from our usual DNA code that it attracts the attention of our immune system, and the new cell gets time and resources to reproduce itself. It unzips the faulty DNA code and uses half of it as a template to build identical twin cancer cells. And those two build another two, and those four build another four and so on. The rogue cancer cell is now generating a tumour of cancer cells undetected by our defenses and in the case of prostate cancer, generating no symptoms to alert us.

Prostate cells with cancer are still prostate cells. They continue to do prostate work like producing PSA. Which is why the blood PSA level rises sharply when an active tumour is present as the rapid cancer cell production exceeds the normal rate of prostate cell replacement.

Once secure and reproducing, prostate cancer cells call for the building of blood vessels (angiogenesis) into their new colony to ensure a supply of oxygen and nutrition to fuel their growth. These new vessels are also the highways for potentially spreading the cancer to other areas of the body.

Simply put, cancer is a malfunction of our cell duplication system which flourishes when undetected by, or exceeds the capacity of, our immune system. There is a lot more to the cancer story than this brief overview. For example, you can 'carry' a cancer gene in your DNA.

Cancer and your DNA

Your DNA coding has the same genes in every cell of your body and you may have inherited genes that make you more likely to develop a specific cancer. Just as women may carry an inherited gene that predisposes them to breast or ovarian cancer, men can inherit a genetic susceptibility for prostate cancer. If your father, uncle, brother or son has been diagnosed with prostate cancer you have an increased genetic risk. Also, if a female relative had breast, ovarian or uterine cancer it is more probable that any prostate cancer you develop will be aggressive.

Having this gene makes it more likely that you will be diagnosed with prostate cancer but it is not a sure thing. There are many factors that determine whether the mutations of your prostate cell DNA will progress to cancer cells able to sustain themselves and reproduce. We have already discussed your immune system and will revisit it later. Other factors include -

1. whether you have ever been a cigarette smoker
2. being overweight or carrying extra abdominal fat
3. how well you regulate your stress hormones
4. how much sugar you consume
5. your alcohol consumption
6. how you cook on the grill
7. how much you worry about stuff (including prostate cancer)

The factors listed may stimulate the prostate cancer gene to switch on as opposed to remaining switched off. Prostate cancer most frequently occurs in older men, yet these men have carried the cancer gene all their lives with no cancer getting hold. What changes over time?

The switch goes on.

For a gene to fulfil its programming, there is a switch to be triggered. This is the science of **epigenetics**: *the study of changes in organisms caused by modification of gene expression rather than alteration of the genetic code itself.*

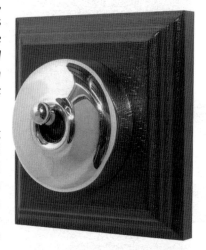

So what regulates this switching mechanism? The switch is a chemical trigger, it responds to chemical changes in your body and when the chemistry is right the cancer switch remains dormant. If the chemistry gets out of balance, the switch may be activated and allow the cancer gene to express itself. Anything that disturbs the normal biochemistry of your inner body workings has the potential to trigger the switch and release the genetic messaging.

Your internal biochemistry can be disturbed by many factors, including chronic inflammation or infection, poor gut function, high levels of stress, hormone fluctuations, exposure to chemicals or radiation, poor sleep patterns, physical illness, poor nutrition or a combination of any of the above. This list is not complete but you can see we have complex systems with many components and processes that all need to work well for us to stay healthy.

SUMMARY

When it comes to prostate cancer development and progression there are two factors you can't change:

- your genetic code (DNA)
- your age (it changes, but in the wrong direction)

There are powerful things you <u>can</u> influence to reduce your risk of developing prostate cancer or having it spread if you are already diagnosed:

- epigenetics - your gene switching system
- immune system resilience - to identify and neutralise DNA mutations
- quality of consumed materials used to resource your cell rebuilding

The strength, persistence and sacrifice needed to make these plays day in and day out is challenging. It will require all your conscious effort. If it was easy, fun or brought immediate rewards you would already be doing it.

Later in this Playbook we will identify the strategies for you to maximise those positive outcomes.

Before that, we will look at Active Surveillance as a treatment option for diagnosed prostate cancer and how it relates to men who may or may not carry a genetic risk gene and have not been diagnosed. Yet.

ACTIVE SURVEILLANCE

Active Surveillance (AS) evolved from 'Watchful Waiting'. You may have come across both terms and wondered if they are different as both relate to delaying curative treatment for prostate cancer.

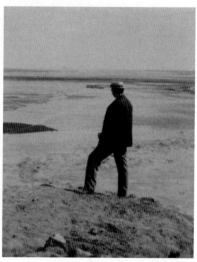

Why bother? What does it matter what we call it? From the medical specialist viewpoint, it probably doesn't matter what <u>we</u> call it. However from your viewpoint, I believe it really matters what <u>you</u> hear it called. Would you prefer to be 'active' in managing your prostate cancer or just 'waiting'?

Watchful waiting

Watchful Waiting suggests a passive mindset as you sit around waiting for your prostate cancer to go rogue. When Watchful Waiting was created there was far less understanding of diagnostic testing, categories of cancer risk and likely progression rates. So waiting was correct - you waited while the urology team did the watching until your diagnostic markers deteriorated to the extent of making curative treatment the better option.

Medical science has turned its collective attention to prostate cancer with increased awareness, funding (thanks Movember) and technology, discovering that all prostate cancers are not equal. Some are fast-growing, aggressive and more prone to causing secondary tumours (metastases). Others are slow-growing, non-aggressive, small volume cancers that remain contained in the prostate gland for years without becoming life threatening. If you are on AS, this is your tumour.

We now have a better understanding of the dynamics of prostate specific antigen (PSA), improved pathology analysis of biopsy samples and huge advances in medical imaging technology (ultrasound and magnetic resonance imaging). This has revealed a spectrum of prostate cancer behaviours and possible outcomes with or without treatment.

As a consequence, your medical team can more confidently predict the likely future of your prostate cancer and make more appropriate recommendations for a treatment plan that not only might extend your life span but also your quality of life for those extra years.

Active Surveillance (or Active Monitoring in the UK) is the upgrade of watchful waiting that takes a more proactive approach to low risk prostate cancer. AS involves regular testing to detect changes in the prostate tumour that may prompt a change in the management plan.

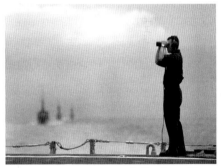

Active Surveillance

The surveillance regime may include any or all of the following -

- PSA levels in the blood, especially the doubling time
- Gleason Scores (grading of likeliness to spread)
- Grade Group System (replacing the Gleason system)
- TNM Score (staging of size and distribution)
- Digital rectal examinations
- Repeat biopsy sampling
- Ultrasound imaging
- Magnetic Resonance Imaging (MRI)
- Other blood test markers (4K, PHI, and those in development)
- DNA analysis

Which is used will depend on the risk analysis for your situation, the preference of your medical team and the medical resources available in your location. The surveillance component asks you to undergo regular testing and re-evaluation until -

- Some other medical condition becomes a higher risk or priority and demands attention
- Your prostate surveillance tests indicate the cancer has become more aggressive or widespread in the prostate gland
- You have become unwell and treating your prostate cancer is no longer an option as you may not tolerate the treatment and/or the side effects of the treatment will decrease your quality of life while giving you no advantage in quantity of life.
- You, your spouse/partner or your physician insist on commencing treatment.

Genetic Risk for Prostate Cancer

This may be your situation - you have a genetic risk courtesy of a primary male relative but have not been diagnosed with prostate cancer. There are two possible reasons for this:

1. You have not undergone any testing
2. You have been tested and no cancer or markers have been detected

Either way, because of your underlying genetic risk you need to remain vigilant in monitoring any changes in your prostate disease markers.

Meanwhile this Playbook offers strategies to reduce the risk of your prostate cancer genetic code being switched on. There is no guarantee, but there is ample evidence that every bit helps to tip the scales toward less chance of mutated cancer cells developing into a prostate tumour.

There are defensive strategies (things to prevent or avoid) as well as offensive strategies (things to initiate, continue or increase).

If you have not tested positive for prostate cancer your motivation to change your lifestyle habits, nutrition, activity, relationships, work-life balance and more will be built on unsteady ground. There is nothing like a diagnosis of cancer to get your attention and prompt some action. The fact you have no evidence of cancer means you will be acting in good faith rather than in fear. You have the the tougher assignment but a lot more to gain.

Two outcomes may play out:

1. You don't develop prostate cancer - a good result that will be impossible to attribute conclusively to these Playbook strategies, but you will be in such excellent health you won't really care.

2. You develop prostate cancer - disappointing (to say the least) and you may regret making all the Playbook changes for no benefit. Get over it. You will arrive for treatment in much better physical shape and health than if you had not made the effort. The fitter you go into treatment, generally the better your recovery. Your heart, immune system, gut, body weight and mind-set will all be in better shape plus you will have demonstrated to yourself that you are prepared to use your strengths and make changes as necessary.

No Genetic Risk for Prostate Cancer

Perhaps this is your situation: you have no known genetic risk factor but are aware of the increasing prevalence of prostate cancer and would like to reduce your overall risk factors. You may have friends or colleagues who have been diagnosed and have seen how difficult life becomes. Having no genetic risk does not mean you cannot develop prostate cancer, only that one of the risk factors is removed.

There are many strategies in this Playbook to help you avoid the prostate cancer path. Even better news, they will also help you avoid the heart disease, dementia, bowel, lung, oesophogeal cancer, diabetes and high blood pressure paths as well.

If you already take a pro-active approach to your health such as watching your eating, getting some regular physical activity and staying in a healthy weight range, there may be some additional strategies or new approaches to help you maintain your enthusiasm for avoiding illness.

Three Strategies

Whether you are already diagnosed, have a known genetic risk, want to keep your prostate healthy or have already undergone treatment there are ways to take control. Each strategic path has numerous options for you to influence the chance of cancer development and/or progression.

The following chapters apply to all three situations, but are written as if you are already diagnosed and have chosen Active Surveillance. Implementing the recommendations will help you reduce your risk profile to avoid a future of active treatment and the life changing side-effects. You can exert your influence by managing your output, your input and your throughput -

Output - the things you do or don't do in terms of physical activity, exercise and training.

Input - what you choose to eat, drink or inhale.

Throughput - your processing systems of thinking, worrying, choosing and behaving.

Each is as important as the others and their effects are not just summative, they are compounding. This means if you address all three areas you don't just add up the benefits, you multiply them because each can increase the potential benefits of the other two.

SUMMARY

Active Surveillance is a legitimate and science-based option for managing low-risk, low-volume prosate cancers.

The surveillance science is well established and your testing cycle will be based on your history, risk, age and health status.

Ignoring the 'Active' element and not following through with lifestyle changes that will reduce your risk of disease progression may increase your chance of needing treatment in the future.

Future treatments may or may not be successful in eradicating your cancer, but either way they expose you to life changing side-effects such as incontinence, erectile dysfunction, fatigue, body temperature fluctuations and pain.

THROUGHPUT

The ancient Greek physicians, the eastern healers and many other 'primitive' health systems understood that the mind and body are linked and interdependent for good health. This remains true as you use all your resources to out-perform prostate cancer. Without the mental tools, control and balance you will struggle to complete the physical program. Your mind and body do their best work when both are aligned on the same path.

Stress

When working with elite athletes, I observed how success was influenced by their ability to manage stress levels. In an Olympic rowing final, there is not 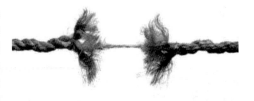 much physical difference between the six teams competing. Each crew has incredible athletes with thousands of hours of rowing drills, weight training, cross training, eating correctly, travel skills and mental preparation.

Their physical and physiological skills and talents are pretty much equal. The crew that wins is often the one that best manages stress levels on the day to allow perfect execution of skills and strategy.

Your goals are more important than sport. You are making improvements to alter your life outcome and to improve your daily capacity to remain continent, potent, employed, active and alive.

You are implementing your high performance strategies during an extremely stressful period in your life: a cancer diagnosis or threat.

Making your best decisions and executing your plan when under peak stress is a hallmark of excellence, not just in sport but in life. Whether it is getting through a job interview, your first solo in a jazz band, asking someone on a date (old school, before technology) or deciding how to best manage your prostate cancer, all will be more successful if you can recognise and manage your stress.

The words 'You have cancer in your prostate' arrive just before you are asked what treatment options you are considering. Most men find this quite stressful and may not hear much of what comes afterwards.

For those of you on Active Surveillance, can you remember the exact moment you heard the word 'cancer' applied to you? Even if you half expected to hear it based on previous conversations, the testing protocols or your family history, there is always a tiny window of hope that anticipates the words: 'We found no cancer'. When reality proves otherwise, everything else becomes foggy, including the specialist explaining the diagnostic pathway and your treatment options. And when you are completely off the planet with unresolved questions and confronting your mortality, hopes and dreams - they ask what you would like to do next.

> A stressed mind does not make clear and rational decisions. Even in mice. Seriously, mice get stressed? Yes, when they are prevented from accessing their food or sleep deprived (sound familiar?). And once stressed, they perform very poorly in a problem solving maze test. In mice with prostate cancer, the stress appears to accelerate the growth and spread of the cancer, driven by increased stress hormone levels.[1]

Navigating his way around PSA results, Gleason scores, biopsy samples, risk profiles and treatment options is the ultimate maze test for a man who is still reeling from the diagnosis. Asking him to choose a logical path at this time is tough and men are often very stressed, uncertain, anxious and frustrated by the process of deciding on a preferred treatment option. He will seek direction from the specialists, opinions from his partner and family and, more recently, appeal for guidance through online support groups.

Despite all this 'help', he must make an important life-changing decision under one, two or many of the following conditions:

- He doesn't fully understand the disease or the treatments being offered
- He is time pressured to make a decision quickly
- There are others to consider in the outcome of his decision
- He doesn't know the financial cost of the choices
- He doesn't know the psychological cost of his choice
- He is trying to trust medical people he has just met
- No one will tell him what is his best option ('It's your decision')
- His final decision may limit his future options for treatment
- His decision will impact his quality of life, but he doesn't know how
- He is apprehensive, fearful and a bit scared
- He is anxious
- He is overwhelmed by new information
- He is not processing information efficiently

Plus his questions that won't go away:

- How will I tell the kids?
- Will my partner think any less of me?
- Will my partner stay the distance?
- Am I sufficiently insured?
- What about work?
- Why didn't I look after myself better?

Once a man makes his decision about treatment, and it doesn't really matter which treatment he selects, his level of distress typically goes down. Making the decision reduces his stress of having to make the decision - who would have thought? His spouse or partner may not experience the same lowering of distress. For them the fear of the future remains strong and they are at risk of depression or anxiety in their own right.[2]

Uncertainty leads to anxiety. All of us prefer certainty so we can prepare accordingly. Anxiety about the treatment decision is somewhat resolved by choosing your treatment, in your case AS. Well done so far.

Decision Regret

The process of decision making has had the stuffing researched out of it and the consensus seems to be that we humans typically make decisions based on imperfect or incomplete information filtered through a series of biased interpretations. Apart from that we're good.

A recent study on emotional (gut response) versus deliberative (brain analysis) decision-making found that those who went with the gut response felt the ultimate decision was more authentic and consistent with their true selves. The group who based their decision on feelings were also more likely to stick to their chosen path.[3] Which is fine as long as it doesn't form a barrier to new information which may need to be factored into a decision review.

Having made your treatment decision, it is incredibly unhelpful if those around you second guess, undermine or question your decision. This includes family, medical team, on-line forum groups, friends, their spouses, employers, work-mates and pretty much anyone else who doesn't have your prostate cancer. No matter how genuine their concerns, it is important your decision is respected rather than subjected to the preferences, doubts, fears, self-interest, bias and assumed expertise of family and friends. Be prepared to defend your position but not with long-winded discussions or arguments. Be concise and explain that you have weighed the options and at this stage AS is the option you have chosen. Remind them that AS is the only option that doesn't come with health-damaging side-effects and leaves open the option for all other treatments in the future should things change. Thank them for their concern and talk about football.

Fighting

The words 'cancer' and 'fight' go together like a pair of comfortable shoes, one is nearly always next to the other. Men speak of 'fighting cancer', 'beating cancer', 'in a battle with cancer' and later they may be spoken of as 'lost his fight with cancer' or was 'beaten in his fight.'

> Cancer bears no animosity to you, it is not fighting you, it is simply a DNA stuff-up. It is not a punishment and it doesn't hate you. It wasn't sent to deprive you of your retirement, relationships and muscle mass.

'Fighting' cancer suggests there must be a winner and a loser. Ideally the cancer will lose but evidence suggests it is often the winner and a very patient winner at that. Perhaps it gains an advantage when the host is exhausted from the fight (the treatments, side-effects, medications, fatigue, frustrations, pain and lack of joy) and no longer has the resources to maintain his fight level.

> Cancer is completely indifferent to you and how you feel about it; you are simply a host organism.
>
> Cancer is your opponent not your enemy. Outplay it.

Physiologically, the stress hormone cortisol is likely to be stimulated by the mental and emotional drivers of 'fighting' or 'battle'. We know cortisol is associated with poorer function of the immune and health systems, so remaining calm rather than angry may improve your chances.

People expect you to fight your cancer and they will be mystified and perhaps uncomfortable if you have opted for AS. They will impose their irrational fears and a fair dose of ignorance as they urge you to seek active treatment, or at least a second opinion (which is code for 'see a doctor who agrees with what I am saying'). This is common in the online patient forums who may mistake their experience for expertise.

The upshot of this is two-fold, firstly you will have to continually justfiy your choice and secondly you will need to develop the resilience and confidence to roll with the prostate cancer as you work to disable it. Most of the cancer management that occurs with AS is hidden. Changes to nutrition, activities, work-life balance, and stress-management are not obvious to others, so they assume you chose not to fight and have given up. Surgery, radiotherapy or hormone therapy (ADT) provide physical evidence of you 'battling' cancer. With AS, you are involved in a covert operation of disruption and sabotage with no obvious signs of a conflict - you are on Black-Ops. You are The Resistance.

The skills and strategies for AS are completely different from those for battle. On Active Surveillance you are playing a long game, trying to maintain a strategic advantage to ensure the game does not end prematurely. You are not trying to win, you are ensuring you don't lose.

Mindfulness

This concept refers to a state where your mind is trained to observe and experience the moment without attaching emotion or significance to it. It is a mental discipline to separate the 'being' from the 'feeling about being'. It sounds simple but is a challenge to master. Personally this is difficult for me, as the idea of taking time to 'do nothing' and focus my mind elsewhere goes against my natural drive to get stuff done and keep busy. Wrong. Mind training is critical for effective health maintenance. Guidance and repeated practice has helped me and I am glad I listened and persisted.

A Canadian study showed an association between mindfulness-based stress reduction and self-reported quality of life in prostate cancer patients.[4] There were measurable improvements in cortisol levels (stress hormone), blood pressure, mood disturbance, inflammatory blood markers and heart rate. These improvements remained for the twelve-month follow up. More research is needed to show the mindfulness training was the cause of their improvement.

Occasionally athletes experience a form slump where they struggle to produce their best skills in game situations. A master coach or psychologist might remark that the player is over-thinking the game rather than just playing it. The internal thinking-noise of perfecting technique, fearing failure, staying confident, worrying about being sent down to a lower division or just embarrassing himself on the field may be stopping him from executing his skills as before. If you ask the player he may tell you that he never used to think about batting, running, catching, shooting, putting, driving, passing, tackling or dribbling: he just did it. His mind was quietly supervising, observing and having fun.

The internal noise and confusion produced by stress can undermine your ability to take in information, analyse the impact, evaluate options and make an informed decision.

This doesn't just apply to sports and athletes. It might be how you went through life at home, work and play until you heard about your cancer and your internal noise level rose dramatically.

The ability to quieten the internal noise and filter the external distractions and confusion is not easy when you are already under stress. Yet this is exactly when it will bring most benefit.

You may need coaching or guidance on how to practice mindfulness or meditation. This can be face-to-face in a class or individual training session or using an online resource or CD-guided sessions. Choose whichever suits your learning style, time management and budget but be sure to keep it going for at least a month or so. As with any new skill it takes time to learn the basics then start to master the content. If you give up because the first couple of sessions were boring, uncomfortable, embarrassing or just too difficult, you are short-changing yourself. This is going to take a while to get the hang of.

If a mental training program doesn't work for you after a month of dedicated effort, you may prefer a combined physical and mental workout. For example, Tai Chi or Yoga where the discipline of following the postures and movements, combined with conscious breathing-control occupies your awareness and provides a haven from your internal noise.[5] As you become more practiced and skilled, you will find it easier to slip into the mental quiet space when you start the routine. Eventually you may be able to generate the mental quietness without even doing the movements or postures. Well done - you are now meditating.

Using preferred music or other tones (e.g. white noise) to block external distractions is a useful tool when learning the skill. Better if the music is without lyrics or you will find yourself singing along in your head. White noise is an unstructured sound that doesn't allow you to hang any meaning to it which might set your mind off in a new direction. White noise apps are plentiful online and some include other sound loops such as a crackling fire, a travelling train, waves washing or traffic noises. This allows you to find the combination that works best for you.

Sleep

Obstructive sleep apnoea may be associated with cancer progression as fragmented sleep and/or hypoxic episodes may impact on immune function, cortisol levels, oxidative stress, inflammation and DNA mutations.[6] This research is not prostate cancer specific and further work is needed to provide more targeted advice.

If you are experiencing fragmented sleep with snoring, frequent cessation of breathing (temporary I hope), excessive daytime tiredness or difficulty with attention or concentration, ask your doctor about undertaking a sleep study. Obtaining a diagnosis and management plan to improve your sleep will equip you with another tool to sabotage and outplay your prostate cancer. It is even more important to follow this up if you are obese, as the combination is a greater health risk for many conditions. Poor sleep doesn't cause cancer, but it weakens your capacity to become cancer-resistant.

THROUGHPUT SUMMARY

Be aware of your mental and emotional load. It will express itself in how you sleep, work, react to people and situations and how you process new information.

Fighting cancer may make you feel like a warrior, but it might be counterproductive. Learn how to outplay your cancer with education, application and mastery. Do not give it the respect of a fight, it is not worthy. Give it no energy at all.

Be open to ideas and activities that previously you thought were soft or mumbo-jumbo new-age time wasters. In that mix might be just the right strategy to help you manage your stress levels.

Seek professional guidance to help you navigate your throughput strategies. You may be the last person to realise how far off the track you have wandered.

Be kind to your support crew, they are on your side.

Throughput References

1. Sazzad H, et al, 2013. Behavioural stress accelerates prostate cancer development in mice. J Clinical Investigation, 123(2):874-886

2. Ulla-Sisko L, et al, 2017. Experiences and psychological distress of spouses of prostate cancer patients at the time of diagnosis and primary treatment. Eur J Cancer Care 27:e12729.

3. Maglio, S. J., & Reich, T. (2018, September 10). Feeling Certain: gut choice, the true self, and attitude certainty. Emotion. Advance online publication. http://dx.doi.org/10.1037/emo0000490.)

4. Carlson L. et al, 2007. One year pre-post intervention follow-up of psychological, immune, endocrine and blood pressure outcomes of mindfulness-based stress reduction (MBSR) in breast and prostate cancer outpatients. Brain Beh and Immunity 21:1038-1049

5. Smith L, et al, 2016. The potential yield of Tai Chi in cancer survivorship. Future Science OA 2(4):F50152

6. Owens R. et al 2016. Sleep and breathing... and cancer? J of Cancer Research, 9(11):921

In the next section we cover your input strategies: what you drink, eat and inhale. Everything you put in your body contributes to your cellular and total health state. Improving input will reinforce your throughput gains as every strategy reinforces the others in the quest to sabotage your cancer.

INPUT

Prostate cancer is an internal problem. The entire process takes place inside your body and never sees the light of day. Which means the only way you can exert any influence over it is through your internal systems and one of the most important is what you are consuming. The materials you put into your body will interact with your prostate gland and cancer. They will ignore, suppress or drive the cancer.

A 2015 study compared the mortality (end-of-life) outcomes of men who had been diagnosed with prostate cancer and then followed one of two dietary patterns: a Western Diet or a Prudent Diet.[1] The study was only interested in their food choices after diagnosis, to evaluate whether what you eat from now on can make a difference to longevity despite already having prostate cancer.

The Prudent diet pattern was characterized by higher intake of vegetables, fruits, fish, legumes and whole grains. The Western diet pattern comprised higher intake of processed meats, high-fat dairy and refined grains.

 The results showed men who adhered to the Western Diet had a higher risk of prostate cancer death in the shorter term than those men on the Prudent Diet. It appears that what you eat makes a significant difference to your disease progression.

The good news is you are in total control of what you choose to consume. Whether it be food, drink, fumes, medication or other chemicals. Equally, you are in control of what you choose not to consume. Here we go.

Smoking

Cigarette smoke contains around 70 carcinogens, the heavy metals cadmium and arsenic, carbon monoxide, particles from the burning fibres and oxidising chemicals. All of which are the last thing your cancer cells need. Well, actually your cancer cells will love it because it keeps your immune system busy trying to preserve all your other cells from the damaging effects of smoking and your prostate cancer wlll take the opportunity to progress.

You may believe smoking benefits your mental or emotional state, helping you cope with the burden of prostate cancer. It is part of your coping strategy. Convincing yourself of this may well make you feel better and give you a sense of control over your situation. It is a shame you are relying on a 'stress management' strategy that has the potential to accelerate the growth and spread of your prostate cancer.

If you smoke, you should stop. Whether it be through nicotine substitution (gum,patches, lozenges, sprays or inhalers), medical or hypnotherapy assistance or just using your stubborn, fierce desire to keep living. Become an ex-smoker from today.

Electronic cigarettes may be an option you consider. These are a new way of maintaining the physical and social rituals around smoking while managing the chemical risks. The long term consequences of e-smoking or vaping have not yet eventuated and the effects on prostate cancer have not been determined. It is likely better than smoking but worse than not smoking. Depending on the brand of e-cigarette (different flavours and ingredients) you may still be inhaling nasty and inflammatory chemicals which could provoke your prostate cancer. Remember your intention to do everything possible to get a good result? Not inhaling toxic fumes is a no-brainer.

If your lungs are not sufficiently important for you to stop smoking remember that it contributes to erectile dysfunction.

Alcohol

This is another input tool commonly used for managing stress and helping us cope with the world. Or so you have convinced yourself.

Enjoyment of the rituals and the social environment lets alcohol become part of our routine. Beer O'Clock, Sundowners, cocktails, wine with dinner become a daily habit. Problem is, your current routine has contributed in some way to developing prostate cancer and if you continue, it may drive the cancer growth. The evidence for alcohol being a causative factor in prostate cancer is not consistent although some research suggests more than three serves of alcohol per day are associated with a 21% higher risk. Other research suggests beer or spirits are more problematic than wine and another suggests the high energy content of alcoholic drinks (calories or kilojoules) contributes to the risk of many cancers through increased body mass (weight gain).

A metastudy (study of all the other studies) in 2017 suggested the occurrence of prostate cancer is not influenced unduly by alcohol consumption, however progression of the disease was more likely to be accelerated by alcohol consumption.[2]

This was confirmed in a Canadian study which looked at post-diagnosis consumption and found increased risk of death from prostate cancer for those men consuming more than eight drinks per week.[3]

> While on AS, limit your alcohol consumption to no more than one serve per day. Try to include two or three alcohol-free days per week to further reduce intake to five or fewer drinks per week.

Your strategy could range from the extreme (remove all alcohol from your home) to a managed risk model. Managed risk includes switching to non-alcoholic drinks at every opportunity, preferably one with no added sugar, caffeine, artificial flavoring, colouring or preservatives.

Are we talking water? Yes! Water is essential for all of your biochemical, physiological and metabolic needs. Every cell in your body needs water to accomplish its work. Each cell is a tiny test-tube of chemical reactions occurring in water. Everything from your nerve conduction to your kidney filtering and from muscle strength to bowel function is affected by your internal water table. Too little and you become dehydrated, sluggish and inefficient. Too much and you pee a lot.

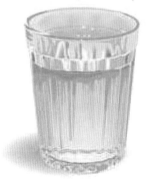

Replacing alcoholic beverages with water is a simple, cheap and healthy way to reduce one of the factors that might be driving your prostate cancer. Depending on your current habit, the cost savings could be huge.

If you find water boring or uninspiring in terms of taste or mouth sensation, try drinking sparkling water or soda water instead. A sort of 'grown up' water. This can get you through social events where you may want to appear more sophisticated and less obviously 'out of the loop'. Or just man up, informing others that you are actively managing your cancer and avoiding alcohol is a simple and powerful way to make a difference.

Finally some good news - if you don't choose to totally give up alcohol, take the opportunity to reward yourself by consuming smaller quantities of higher quality. Five days with only one drink and two days alcohol free per week is taking control and reducing your cancer fuel.

Coffee

While on the topic of commonly consumed beverages, the planet-wide coffee boom needs to be discussed. Coffee gets a lot of good and bad press - it can increase productivity, may help manage chronic pain and improve some cardiovascular disease markers. On the negative side it can raise blood pressure, aggravate inflammatory joint pain, increase urinary frequency and interfere with normal sleep patterns.

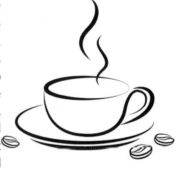

Research related to prostate cancer suggests there is some protection afforded by compounds in coffee that can reduce the risk of lethal prostate cancer.[4] Men who drink six or more cups per day are most protected and the effect decreases with consumption rates. More importantly, the effect is equal for normal and decaffeinated coffee. Meaning the stimulant effect can be avoided as the prostate protection is delivered by one or more of the other hundred or so compounds in coffee. Note also that pesticides and herbicides may be used in coffee production and can remain in the finished product, so it may be wise to choose an organically produced brand of coffee to reduce your agricultural chemical exposure.

Inflammatory Foods

There is plenty of research suggesting that the level of inflammation in your body will affect your health. We are not talking about the short term inflammation from a cut, sprain or impact injury where there is redness, swelling, local pain and increased temperature. That type of inflammation is a response to new tissue damage and triggers the next stage of healing. Having done its job the inflammatory response subsides within a day or so. We are more interested in the chronic type.

Your body has a baseline level of inflammation throughout the tissues and fluids. This is a product of normal cell activity, the processing of waste products and elimination of toxic substances, dead cell debris and so on. Your inflammatory markers can be detected during a blood test to determine if they fall within the normal range.

Prolonged elevated levels of inflammatory markers indicate higher risk of several illnesses including cardiovascular disease (atherosclerosis), arthritis, osteoporosis, neurological diseases, asthma, gut diseases and many cancers.

One of the factors that strongly influences your inflammatory level is what you choose to eat. Some foods tend to increase inflammation while others are neutral or may reduce the inflammation levels.

Each of us has our own built-in inflammation balancing systems, and we respond differently to different foods. For example, those with coeliac disease have a strong inflammatory response to gluten in food. For others, a particular fruit (e.g. tomato or avocado) may trigger inflammatory skin rashes.

Your prostate will not immediately react to the food you eat but it will be exposed to the components once they are absorbed in the gut and circulated in the blood stream. If your food input increases your inflammatory levels your prostate will be affected. Inflammation anywhere in your body will be detected by your immune system whose job is to resolve it so normal cellular function can resume. Multiple sites of inflammation tax the resources of your immune response leaving weakened defences to deal with immature cancer cell mutations in your prostate.

There are many anti-cancer and anti-inflammatory diets in the press and on the web. Some are trying to sell you their 'miracle' product, supplement or program. Others are promoted by people who have had good results or want to be part of a movement. While these are interesting and often convincing, they may not be based on scientific fact and valid research.

My professional training bias is toward the scientific, medical and research information. However, we all respond differently, and if you don't get the results you hope for, try other strategies. You may find the right nutritional balance that works for you even though it lacks scientific support. Be sure to keep your medical team informed about what you are taking or any changes in your diet. This is especially important if you are taking any prescription medication where the efficacy of that drug may be diluted or amplified by changes to your diet or supplements.

Reducing overall inflammatory load is supported by research using men who had raised PSA levels and a negative biopsy for prostate cancer. The men who used aspirin or a non-steroidal anti-inflammatory medication had a lower incidence of prostate cancer on subsequent biopsy than those men who did not use the medication. The effect was slight but noticeable.[5]

Lowering inflammation using medication exposes men to the side-effects of the drugs themselves. It would be safer to reduce inflammation through food choices where the only side-effects might be weight loss, improved mood, reduced cholesterol levels and improved bowel function. Pretty good side-effects.

If you are prescribed anti-inflammatory medication for a treatable condition, please follow your doctor's guidance. You can still adjust your food choices to reduce your inflammatory load while on medication to gain even more benefit without any extra risk.

Before listing low-inflammatory foods to increase in your diet (offensive strategy) and the high-inflammatory foods to reduce (defensive strategy) get ready to be disappointed on two fronts. Firstly, I will not be claiming there are any superfoods that will cure prostate cancer, and secondly you may have to change your palate preferences, food preparation techniques (cooking) and how you relate to your food intake. From now on, look at food as medicine. and make this a primary decision-maker about what and how much to eat.

You may need to change domestic patterns and start contributing to food selection and preparation. This is your self-efficacy at work. This is the agreement you made when you decided to work around the cancer without active treatment. Work together with your partner at home to improve your knowledge and skills and develop a pro-active approach to shopping, preparing, cooking and enjoying a new way of eating.

The table below lists low-inflammatory foods as supported by nutritional research. You may already know some of them, which is great but there maybe others that are more powerful and give you more choice in your diet. The second column lists the foods to reduce, as they are more likely to provoke inflammation. The list is not exhaustive, but provides a useful starting point to modify your eating habits.

Good Choices	Poor Choices
Dark leafy greens (kahle, spinach)	Processed meats
Dark berries, cherries, grapes	Sugary drinks (soda pop, juices)
Cruciferous Vegetables (broccoli, bok, cabbage, Brussels sprouts)	Trans fats (fried food)
Beans, lentils	White bread and pasta
Avodado, coconut	Gluten (where sensitive)
Olives and extra virgin olive oil	Soybean oil, vegetable oils
Walnuts, pistachios, almonds, Brazil nuts	Processed snack food (chips, crackers)
Turmeric	Sweet desserts
Cold water fish (salmon, sardines)	Excess alcohol
Dark chocolate & red wine (moderate)	Excess carbohydrate (quantity)

Take a sticky note and write *'Page 36'* then put it on your refrigerator door. This is your secret reminder to step up and make consistently strong decisions in the kitchen. Every time you see the note you will recall the reason for making input changes. Revisit this chapter when it gets difficult, and refresh your determination to keep going. You are not in a fight, you are managing this cancer with smart decisions and persistence.

Sugar

Sugar is sometimes described as a cancer driver or providing fuel for cancer but the direct evidence for this relationship is still evolving and is much contested by manufacturers of sugar-dense food and drink. Researchers have established that higher dietary levels of added sugar increase the body's chronic inflammation level.[6] Other studies show a direct link between that inflammation and a higher risk of prostate cancer onset and progression.[7] This domino effect clearly indicates that reducing the consumption of added sugar in your diet is an important strategy to undermine prostate cancer.

Sugar is present in many foods in their natural and processed states, including fruits and vegetables, where it is consumed in proportion with accompanying fibre, vitamins, minerals and other nutrient partners which can help neutralise the oxidative stress (see more on page 40). This sugar consumption is limited by how much of these bulkier foods you can eat. When sugar is added during the manufacture of food/drink or added at the point of serving, the concentration is often much higher than the natural sugar occurrence in food. This higher level of sugar increases the inflammatory load throughout the body with increased oxidative stress and potential DNA damage.

One study lists the sources of added sugar as soft drinks (sodas), milkshakes, punch, fruit drinks, sugar or honey added to tea or coffee, sweet desserts, cakes, cookies, pies, pastries, chocolate, candy, syrups, ice-cream and puddings[1]. There is your list of foods to progressively eliminate and avoid as you start to starve your cancer.

Sugar is a hidden ingredient in many processed foods, so read the ingredient lists on products to discover where sugar ranks (highest percentages are listed first) and the nutritional information/facts panel to see how many kilojoules/calories and carbohydrates (they break down to sugar)are contained. Some countries express these values as a percentage of recommended daily intake (e.g. USA and Canada), others as a quantity per recommended serving size and/or quantity in a standard amount (e.g. Australia, UK and New Zealand). Both styles allow a comparison between products to inform your purchase decision. For more information on interpreting nutritional labels search your government health or food safety sites.

For best damage control, it is recommended to avoid all sweetened, sugary drinks and not add sugar to tea, coffee or cereals. Or anything else. Alcohol does not disable sugar so if you prefer cola or sweet mixers with your spirits, switch to unflavoured, unsweetened carbonated or mineral water. And consider taking the virgin option - leave out the alcohol.

You will need to be constantly vigilant as the food scientists and marketers of the world are very creative in trying to slip sugar past your defences. You have more to gain by denying them, so move beyond your sugar cravings and re-train your taste palate to enjoy all inputs without added sugar. You will know you have succeeded when any inadvertent exposure to high sugar will pain your teeth and give you a headache. Well done.

Kilojoules, Calories and Energy Density

The total energy content of your entire dietary intake may be an important influence on prostate tumour growth. Research from the University of Illinois using animal models showed carbohydrate, lipid (fat) or total diet restriction inhibited prostate cancer growth to a similar level as did androgen deprivation treatment.[8] Your energy requirements will depend on your activity level, metabolic rate, muscularity, glucose utilisation efficiency and other factors. If you decide to try this strategy I recommend you do so under professional guidance with your physician or nutritionist. This is to ensure any health risks do not outweigh the benefits.

A less extreme approach is to identify foods you currently consume that are energy dense but nutritionally light. These foods will be high in sugar or animal fats but low in vitamins, proteins, minerals and trace elements. Examples include alcoholic drinks, processed snack and convenience foods, fast-food, deep-fried anything, ice-cream and other sweet desserts, candy, cookies, commercial bakery goods and sweet fizzy drinks. If you are wondering what is left to eat, keep reading.

Vegetables

Unsurprisingly, fresh and well prepared vegetables are generally a healthy food. Nutritionists recommend eating at least five servings of vegetables every day and to eat a mix of colours - green, red, orange, yellow; and a mix of textures - leafy and crunchy.

> Researchers from University of Washington found men consuming 28 or more servings of vegetables per week had a 35% reduced risk of prostate cancer compared with those eating fewer than 14 servings.[9] Those who included at least three servings of cruciferous vegetables upped their risk reduction to 41%.

Sounds simple: 28 servings of vegetables across your 21 meals per week. You may think you already do this most weeks. Try keeping a food diary of everything (and how much) you consume for a few weeks and see how many times you hit this target. Or think back over the last few days (less reliable). And if you are not achieving the 28 serves per week, why do you think that is? Choose from the following possible reasons:

1.   Don't enjoy eating vegetables (boring, tasteless)
2.   Can't be bothered preparing them (peeling, washing, cooking)
3.   Never have vegetables in the house (don't buy them)
4.   All of the above

These reasons may be personal or could apply to your partner or family. Either way, the three reasons listed above could stem from the following knowledge or experience gaps:

1.   You don't know how to prepare vegetables in a tasty and attractive way

2. You are uncomfortable, unwelcome or unskilled in the kitchen
3. You get confused or overwhelmed by the choices in stores

All of these gaps can be overcome to maximise the sabotage of your prostate cancer. Devote your energy toward acquiring food knowledge and skills to help disrupt your tumour growth. Resist the easy path of 'why bother' or 'too late now' or 'I might as well eat what I like and enjoy my remaining time'.

If you can't get past this huge barrier of how to get more vegetables into your daily diet you are going to hate the next section on physical activity. In fact, you probably should hand this book onto someone who will actually make an effort and change his basic attitudes and behaviours to improve his health. Better still, if you have a son, give it to him as he has a genetic predisposition to prostate cancer and if he follows this advice before diagnosis he may never need to seek it out after a diagnosis. If you get my drift.

Identify your vegetable habits and barriers to change. Then make the necessary changes in small steps. Don't try and change everything at once; that is too big a job especially given your stress situation.

Seek advice from nutrition professionals who can offer a solution that works around lack of knowledge or skills. Do a cooking class, talk with your fruit vendor, go online for ideas, recipes and lessons, try new foods when dining out and ask how they get their vegetables so tasty (probably add butter). Or identify a friend with excellent vegetable cooking skills and ask him/her for help. Learn how to enjoy preparing food in the kitchen, all you need is some knowledge and confidence. Just like everything else you do. None of us was born knowing how to cook.

Cruciferous Vegetables

These are the big-league vegetables when it comes to sabotaging cancer. In fact the word 'cruciferous' means 'bad-ass to cancer'. Or something like that.

> 'High consumption of vegetables, particularly cruciferous, is associated with a reduced risk of prostate cancer.' [9]

These vegetables have a common flower structure of four petals from their stem that forms a sort of cross. The other thing they have in common is a generous dose of anti-oxidant nutrition that damps down inflammation throughout your body. However, they are often an acquired taste as you improve your food preparation skills to make these vegetables tasty, attractive and a go-to strategy for cancer suppression.

Here is a list of cruciferous vegetables -

Cabbage (inc. Chinese)	Broccoli	Cauliflower
Brussels Sprouts	Bok Choi	Arugula / Rocket
Artichokes	Collard Greens	Daikon
Radish	Rutabaga	Turnips
Mustard (seeds & leaves)	Watercress	Horseradish

You can vary your cruciferous intake as you become better at preparing and enjoying them. Check the range available at your local store and see what they have in season, they might even have some recipe cards on hand to get you started. If no local supplier exists, you could try growing your own.

Lycopene

This is a food component found in tomatoes that has a role in reducing DNA damage due to oxidative stress. As your cells convert food to energy it can create unstable molecules that have unpaired electrons (free radicals). Until they find another molecule to accept or donate an electron (unradicalise) they can cause cellular damage, including to DNA. When the free radicals are generated from oxygen molecules it is called **oxidative stress**. Free radicals are a normal result of your cell activities throughout the body and are disabled (buffered) by anti-oxidants produced internally (e.g. vitamin D) or ingested as part of your diet (e.g. vitamin C). When you are unwell, stressed, eating poorly, fatigued, not sleeping or experiencing some other out-of-balance situation, the production of free radicals overwhelms your capacity to neutralise them. Your immune system is inhibited by this imbalance and cancer cells may escape detection and destruction.[10]

Lycopene decreases the aggressive potential of prostate cancer by inhibiting the development of blood vessels into the tumour.[11]

Lycopene concentration is low in fresh tomatoes but much higher in tomato concentrate products such as tomato ketchup, sauce or paste. Use them as condiments or bases in other dishes rather than eaten alone. What you add them to is important and a poor choice will negate any lycopene advantage.

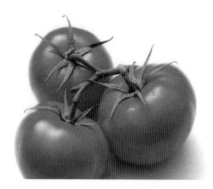

If you plan to eat pizza four times per day to get lycopenes from the tomato paste, any advantage is cancelled out by the processed meat, cheese, beers and red wine. Sorry.

Lycopene-rich products are only as healthy as the food they accompany. So be smart in your choices, for example, substitute a vegetarian pizza for the meat-lovers and use high-fibre pasta with a lean-mince for spaghetti bolognese. Small changes make a difference when repeated consistently.

Or from left-field, make a pizza using cauliflower for the base, add the tomato paste, grilled sweet potato (yam), red capsicum (pepper), onion, garlic, fresh spinach on top, sprinkle with pizza cheese mix and olive oil. Into the oven and you have a low carb, meat-free, lycopene enriched, vegetable laden pizza to have with your mineral water or low alcohol beer. Guilt free and delicious cancer-busting pizza (Google: 'cauli pizza').

Garlic & Onion

While on the topic of pizza, a recent study suggested garlic and onion may reduce prostate cancer risk, but the benefits did not occur if the garlic was taken as a supplement (pill or powder) rather than a whole food.[12] Again, the importance of organic (low chemical load) and fresh (local) garlic or onions is stressed and remember to use them in healthy, anti-inflammatory, anti-oxidant rich dishes to maximise the value.

Nuts

If you expect me to make the obvious link between nuts and prostate cancer you will have to wait until the end of this section. Happily the link is postive and not just for Brazil nuts. A study in the New England Journal of Medicine[13] found that people who ate a handful of nuts every day were less likely to die from any cause when compared with those who never consumed nuts.[13] There is more research needed, but the consumption of nuts has been linked to reducing inflammation and oxidative stress, protecting against diabetes, improving blood pressure and cardiovascular disease and reducing the onset, spread and recurrence of cancer.[14]

While Brazil nuts are the stand out (possibly because they are a seed, not a nut), almonds, pistachios, walnuts, pecans and peanuts (a legume) all have anti-inflammatory properties. Especially if eaten with their skin on, as most of the good stuff is in the skin to protect the core of the nut from oxidation as it waits to germinate and grow a tree.

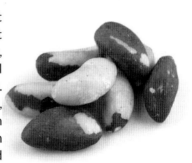

There is little evidence to support that 'activating' of nuts (pre-soaking and then slow-drying them) provides any additional nutritional benefit beyond actually eating the nut. Remember, once you chew and swallow it, the nut is now soaking internally as it's component ingredients are broken down for absorption into your body. It doesn't get more activated than that.

For more on 'activating your nuts' check my book 'Prostate Recovery MAP - Men's Action Plan' for those recovering after treatment for their prostate cancer (www.prostaterecoverymap.com). I couldn't resist.

Dairy Foods

This group includes milk, cheese, butter, yoghurt and other cows' milk products. There is a lot of nutritional research on dairy intake and cardiovascular health, obesity and gut irritability with less addressing the relationship with prostate cancer.

One study looked at dairy consumption after diagnosis of localised prostate cancer and found consuming more than three serves per day was associated with an increased risk of prostate-specific and all-cause mortality.[15] Whether the dairy was low or high fat content made no difference to the outcome of the prostate cancer mortality, however those men on high-fat dairy had a higher all-cause mortality than those who chose low-fat options. Reducing your total disease burden is a valuable strategy to free more of your internal resources (energy, immune system capacity, free radical buffering) to make life difficult for prostate cancer.

Here are some guidelines for dairy consumption -

1. Don't add milk to coffee, tea or alcoholic drinks. Drink it black or neat.
2. Use low fat milk on cereal. And everything else.
3. Avoid cream in or on anything. Push it aside if served with dessert.
4. Reduce or avoid butter on your toast, bagels, sandwiches.
5. Use non-dairy 'milks' such as almond, oat, rice, coconut or soy.
6. Consume yoghurt in moderation for the pro-biotic bacteria and only the non-sweetened (natural or otherwise), lower fat options.

These options are all achievable. The only barrier will be a lack of determination and planning. Plus peer pressure, life-long habits and lack of support at home. Be ready for all these and rise above them.

Meat, Fish, Poultry and Eggs

Research from the Harvard School of Public Health on diet and prostate cancer progression showed men with higher-grade prostate cancer were more likely to be the higher consumers of red meat and/or eggs.[16] Disease progression was not related to intake of red meat, fish or eggs, however a high intake of poultry was associated with a reduced rate of progression. They concluded that substituting 30g of poultry or fish for 30g/day of unprocessed red meat was associated with significantly lower risk of cancer recurrence.[16]

They also noted that eating well-done red meat added significantly to the risk of developing advanced prostate cancer. So it is not just the meat but how it is grilled.

'Lower intakes of red meat and well-done red meat and higher intakes of poultry and fish are associated with lower risk of high grade and advanced prostate cancer and reduced recurrence risk, independent of stage and grade'.[16]

Another study concluded that fish consumption didn't make much of a difference in whether we get prostate cancer, but it makes a significant difference in the likelihood of that cancer metastasizing to other tissues or organs.[17] Less chance of moving from Stage 2 to Stages 3 or 4.

The take away message is simple, no matter what your PSA or Gleason Score you are less likely to drive the progression of your cancer if you reduce red meat (especially well-done) and substitute white meat or fish. If you review the table on inflammatory foods (page 35) you will see a common theme.

Soy Foods

Variation in the prevalence of prostate cancer internationally has led to investigating any possible role of soy bean food products in the diet. Food such as tofu, edamame, miso, soy milk and tempeh.

The reseach has brought mixed results as to whether soy products offer protection or increase cancer aggression. This may reflect the different ways of measuring soy levels (estimated intake, circulating levels in blood flow versus bound in the prostate gland) and whether the soy products are unfermented (e.g. edamame, soy milk, tofu) or fermented (e.g. miso, tempeh, natto, tamari).

An extensive review of these studies drew the following conclusions[18] -

- total soy food consumption is associated with decreased prostate cancer risk
- Once bound in the prostate cells, soy-based isoflavones may reduce PSA levels and inhibit prostate carcinogenesis
- Fermented soy products were more effective than unfermented in reducing prostate cancer risk.
- Tofu appears to offer a significant protective association

The researchers also pointed out that more definitive information is required and geographical variation in research findings makes it difficult to be conclusive.[18] Suggestions if you are on AS are:

> - Moderate levels of soy foods are safe and may offer protection.
> - Fermented soy may be more effective.
> - If you don't currently eat soy products, start adding them to your diet.
> - If you do currently eat soy products you can safely continue.
>
> *Soy products are just another piece in the nutrition jigsaw, not a miracle treatment for prostate cancer.*

Dietary Supplements

Down the rabbit hole we go. There are many opinions, anecdotes, sales pitches, advertisers, marketers and health professionals (real or pretend) who claim to know which dietary supplements are good for prostate cancer. Or bad for prostate cancer. Much of this material is unsubstantiated by scientific investigation in studies where other factors are sufficiently controlled so as to allow outcomes to be reliably attributed to a specific supplement. So this discussion operates under two fundamental rules:

1. Supplements must not increase your health risk in their own right or substitute for proven treatments (do no harm).
2. You will need to evaluate the cost versus potential benefit for your individual circumstances (do no financial harm).

Supplements are often promoted as being 'natural' which sounds comforting and safe. However, if you are taking a supplement in pill, liquid, gel or vapor form it is not natural. It is a product derived from some source to mimic the action of the natural product that you would normally absorb from your food or fluid intake. It has come through a production process in a factory somewhere using ingredients from somewhere else and made to a price in order to sell in the supplement market.

Some products also arrive with endorsements from health professionals, sporting or other celebrities. Rarely are these endorsements given for no personal gain. They may be shareholders, creators or paid influencers who all have some skin in the game and a commercial reason for you to purchase their product. Truth is, every branded product has a commercial drive for you to purchase and many claims are made about their products. To avoid the same charge, I won't be recommending brands or proprietorial names. You may have to do some research based on the following generic information.

> *Dietary supplements are not meal replacements or antidotes for poor food choices.*
>
> *That is why they are called 'supplements'.*

Multi Vitamins & Multi Minerals

These products claim to ensure you receive all your necessary vitamins and minerals for optimal heatlh. They will tell you about the range of ingredients and the purity of manufacture. They will associate themselves with sports teams or athletes, with many of the former being possibly unaware of the sponsorship or the product, yet happy to benefit from the association.

Generally they do no harm, possibly because they contain so little of any one vitamin or mineral that they may not actually deliver an effective dose. There is a compromise when producing a multi-product and targeting the lower price range: put everything in, but not too much. My preference is to use the highest priced product I can afford, and read the ingredient list to ensure the quantity and range of the key ingredients meets my health needs now and into the future.

I recently compared a low and a high priced multi-vitamin and found the cheaper product was actually more expensive on a 'dollar per microgram' for many key nutrients. One product had up to four times the amount of Vitamins C, B1, B2, B3, B6, B12 and E among its more extensive ingredient list compared with the other, yet was only 2.5

times more expensive. The cheaper brand spent a lot on TV advertising and athlete brand ambassadors, the other invested in quality products.

How long do you need to stay on a supplement program? A very large Chinese study established that after 5 years of taking supplements, benefits continued for up to an additional 10 years with no further supplementation.[19] So you should take them until around 8 years before you die. Or hedge your bets and just keep taking them if you feel your supplements comply with both rules on page 45.

Selenium

Selenium is a naturally occuring trace element that has proven anti-inflammatory, anti-carcinogenic (DNA repair) and other health benefits. As regards prostate cancer, an optimal level of selenium appears to offer some protection.[20,21] If a man is selenium deficient an increase in his diet or through a supplement is advised. However if he has a normal level and takes a supplement it may increase his prostate cancer risk. Too little or too much selenium is not ideal.

Short term exposure to selenium results in a higher level in your blood stream which rises and falls based on what you have eaten recently. Long term exposure is measured in your fingernails which is a more reliable measure of your selenium absorption over an extended period.

The original source of selenium is the soil where it is absorbed into plants which are then eaten either by us directly or by other animals. If the soil has low selenium content you will have to eat more of the plants to get the same levels. Eating livestock provides a more consistent level of selenium as they tend to concentrate it in their organ and muscle meats.

The western diet generally has adequate selenium for an adult and, if your selenium is in the normal range, supplementation may be ill-advised.

The table on the next page lists foods rich in selenium (in descending order). The list is not complete and only provides a guide.

• Brazil Nuts (way out in front)	• Turkey (roast)
• Tuna (grilled)	• Beef liver
• Sardines (canned, in oil, drained)	• Chicken
• Ham (roast)	• Brown rice (long grain)
• Prawns / Shrimp	• Egg (hard boiled)
• Macaroni (enriched)	• Oatmeal (cooked with water)
• Beef steak (roast)	• Spinach

Omega-3 Fatty Acids

Omega-3 fatty acids are often mentioned as a beneficial element of fish in your diet and also available as a supplement, for example in fish-oil. Their effect is primarily anti-inflammatory and thus may reduce cancer progression. A strong study in Canada looked at the Omega-3 fatty acid within the prostate tissue using a sample taken during biopsy and monitored any subsequent cancer progression.[22] All the subjects were on Active Surveillance. While their research suggested omega-3 supplements offered 'a potential protective effect' on prostate cancer carcinogenesis, this was a side-bar from their main study. Their results showed marine omega-3 fatty acids (from fish) seem to be protective against progression of prostate cancer. Meaning, Omega-3 fatty acids may not prevent you getting prostate cancer, but they may reduce the progression of the cancer. Studies measuring Omega-3 levels using food questionnaires, blood plasma levels or red cell membrane measures have been less conclusive about this protective relationship, suggesting the Omega-3s need to get into the prostate tissues and stay long term as would happen with eating oily fish regularly over a long period.

Another study showed men with prostate cancer tended to have a higher level of Omega-3 fatty acids in their blood but it is unclear if this was from diet changes or supplements taken since diagnosis.[23] A 2017 systematic review of 44 studies concluded there was 'insufficient evidence to suggest a relationship between marine Omega-3 fatty acid intake and risk of prostate cancer'.[24]

You may receive varied advice from different health professionals (and other well-intentioned advisors) depending on what research they have read. You are entitled to be confused, and the only reassurance I can offer is firstly, Omega-3 fatty acids do not appear to increase PSA levels in your blood, suggesting they are not irritating the prostate beyond the 'normal' cancer growth.[25] Secondly, the anti-inflammatory benefits of Omega-3 fatty acids extend beyond your prostate and may offer health benefits elsewhere.

If you choose to take fish oil supplements be sure to advise your medical team and use moderate quantities of quality products.

Vitamin C

Also known as ascorbic acid, vitamin C is an anti-oxidant effective in reducing DNA damage or mutations and has a cancer prevention effect against carcinogens. Vitamin C cannot be manufactured in our bodies so must be ingested through diet or supplementation. A very large study looking only at dietary vitamin C through food (mainly fruit and vegetables) showed a 9% protection effect against prostate cancer for each 150 mg/day consumed. A similar effect for vitamin C supplements was not reported.[26]

Including vitamin C enriched fruits and vegetables such as citrus fruits, berries, tomatoes, capsicum, broccoli, broccolini, sprouts and guavas in your regular diet is highly recommended, especially those with anti-inflammatory properties (usually low acidity).

Cooking foods can reduce their vitamin C levels before you eat them. Ideally, eat them raw but for those that need cooking it is recommended to cook them at a low heat in small amounts of water for short periods. Microwaved or pressure cooked vegetables retain vitamin C more so than boiling or steaming. Broccoli lightly pan-fried in a small amount of butter or olive oil is not only delicious but more nutritious. Don't cook the goodness out of your vegetables.

Vitamin D

Results for prostate cancer and vitamin D are mixed in terms of the risk of getting the cancer. Some studies say it offers protection, others say not and others can't be sure. This may be irrelevant in your case as you have already been diagnosed. There is even less research on vitamin D supplementation for prevention of cancer progression. A study of men on Active Surveillance showed a one year program of vitamin D supplementation reduced disease progression to only 34% of subjects versus 63% in the control group, a reduction of almost half. Yet there was no effect on PSA levels.[27]

Vitamin D does have benefits for calcium absorption (retaining bone structure) and some brain benefits (memory and attention). As it does no harm in regards to prostate cancer it may still be on your list.

Vitamin E

A fat-soluble antioxidant occurring in many foods, vitamin E may help with immune function and DNA repair. Too much vitamin E appears to increase your risk of prostate cancer and it is recommended that men get their vitamin E from food rather than supplements, aiming for a minimum intake of 15 mg/day and staying well below a maximum of 1000 mg/day.

Foods high in vitamin E include spinach, tomato sauce (ketchup), capsicum, avocado, eggs, sardines, tuna, almonds, peanut butter, brazil nuts and cereal grains.

Turmeric

This spice has an active component, curcumin, shown to have anti-inflammatory properties and an ability to induce prostate cancer cell death.[28]

Dried, powdered turmeric can be added to salads or cooked dishes such as curries or stews. The ground root can be steeped for a tea, and sweetened with honey to offset the bitterness. A daily intake of around half a teaspoon per day is recommended which can be spread across several meals. Consuming turmeric in combination with black pepper increases the curcumin bioavailability, often seen in Chai tea blends.

Turmeric can also be taken as a supplement. Excessive intake may cause gastric pain and irritation. Avoid turmeric supplements if you are taking diabetic or blood thinning medication.

INPUT SUMMARY

We have covered a lot of information in this Input chapter. There is much to consider and evaluate in terms of what you could do, should do and will do.

The following check list provides a range of interventions which you can tick off as you succeed with them. Not just try them, but make them part of your everyday health related behaviours.

- ☐ Cease smoking
- ☐ Ensure alcohol consumption is within recommended daily levels
- ☐ Have at least two alcohol-free days per week
- ☐ Switch to decaf coffee with no added milk or sugar
- ☐ Learn to prepare anti-inflammatory foods in an appealing and tasty way
- ☐ Become fluent in Nutritional Information or Facts Panels
- ☐ Put a sticky note with 'Page 36' on the fridge door
- ☐ Eliminate added sugar and reduce 'hidden' sugar in your diet
- ☐ Buy, prepare and eat cruciferous vegetables 4 times per week
- ☐ Eat a handful of nuts, especially Brazil nuts, each day as a snack
- ☐ Use only small quantities of high quality dairy products
- ☐ Don't overcook the small amounts of red meat you consume
- ☐ Substitute white meat or fish for red meat at every opportunity
- ☐ Learn to love tofu (seriously, it can be done)
- ☐ Improve your diet before relying on supplements
- ☐ Find ways to include turmeric in your eating plan

Input References

1.   Yang M, et al, 2015. Dietary patterns after prostate cancer diagnosis in relation to disease-specific and total mortality. Cancer Prev Research 8:545-551

2.   Brunner C, et al, 2017. Alcohol consumption and prostate cancer incidence and progression: a Mendeliean randomisation study. Int J of Cancer 140:75-85.

3.   Farris M et al, 2018. Post-diagnosis alcohol intake and prostate cancer survival: a population-based cohort study. Int J of Cancer 143:253-262.

4.   Wilson K, et al, 2011. Coffee consumption and prostate cancer risk and progression in the health professionals follow-up study. J National Cancer Inst. 103(11):876-884

5.   Vidal A. et al, 2014. Aspirin, NSAIDs and risk of prostate cancer. Results from the REDUCE study. Cancer Prev Research 8(10 Suppl):nrPR04

6.   Miles F. et al. 2018. Concentrated sugars and incidence of prostate cancer in a prospective cohort. Br J Nutrition 120(6):703-710.

7.   Sfanos K & De Marzo A, 2012. Prostate cancer and inflammation: the evidence. Histopathology 60(1):199-215.

8.   Mukherjee P, 1999. Energy intake and prostate tumor growth, angiogenesis, and vascular endothelial growth factor expression. J National Cancer Inst. 91(6):512-23

9.   Cohen J, et al, 2000. Fruit and vegetable intakes and prostate cancer risk. J National Cancer Inst. 92(1):61

10. Lanwen C, et al, 2001. Oxidative DNA damage in prostate cancer patients consuming tomato sauce-based entrees as a whole-food intervention. J. National Cancer Institute.93(24):1873

11. Ke Zu, et al, 2014. Dietary lycopene, angiogenesis and prostate cancer: a prospective study. J. National Cancer Institute. 106(2):djt430 doi:10.1093/jnci/djt430

12. Nicastro H, Ross S & Milner J, 2015. Garlic and onions: their cancer prevention properties. Cancer Prev Research 8:181-189

13. Fillon, M. 2014. News: Nuts may lower cancer risk. J. Nat. Cancer Inst. 106(4).

14. Falasca M, et al 2014. Cancer chemoprevention with nuts. J Nat Cancer Inst. 106(9):dju238 doi:10.1093

15. Yang, M et al, 2015. Dairy intake in relation to disease-specific and total mortality after prostate cancer diagnosis. J Can Prev Research, 8(10 Suppl):nrA32

16. Szymanksi K, et al, 2010. Fish consumption and prostate cancer risk: a review and meta-analysis. Am. Journal of Clinical Nutrition 92:1223-33.

17. Wilson K et al, 2016. Meat,fish, poultry and egg intake at diagnosis and risk of prostate cancer progression. J Cancer Prevention Research. 9(12):933-41.

18. Applegate C, et al, 2018. Soy consumption and the risk of prostate cancer: an updated systematic review and meta-analysis. Nutrients 10,40;doi:10.3390

19. Wang S, et al, 2018. Effects of nutrition intervention on total and cancer mortality: 25-year post-trail follow up of the 5-year Linxian nutrition intervention trial. J. National Cancer Inst. 110(11):djy043

20. Christensen M. 2014. Selenium and prostate cancer prevention: what next - if anything? Cancer Prev Research 7(8):781-5

21. Kristal A, et al, 2014. Baseline selenium status and effects of selenium and vitamin e suplementation on prostate cancer risk. J Natl Cancer Inst. 106(3)

22. Moreel X, et al, 2014. Prostatic and dietary omega-3 fatty acids and prostate cancer progression during active surveillance. Cancer Prev. Res. 7(7):767-76

23. Brasky T.M. et al, 2013. Plasma phospholipid fatty acids and prostate cancer risk in the SELECT trial. J National Cancer Inst. 105(15):1132-41.

24. Aucoin, M. et al, 2017. Fish-derived omega-3 fatty acids and prostate cancer: a systematic review. Integ. Cancer Therapies 16(1):32-62

25. DeFina L. et al, 2016. Association between omega-3 fatty acids and serum prostate specific antigen. Nutrition & Cancer 68(1):58-62

26. Xiao-Yan Bai, et al, 2015. Association between dietary vitamin C intake and risk of prostate cancer: a meta-analysis involving 103,658 subjects. J of Cancer 6(9):913-921

27. Marshall D, et al. 2012 Vitamin D3 supplementation at 4000iU/d for one year results in a decrease of positive cores at repeat biopsy in subjects with low-risk prostate cancer under active surveillance. J Clin. Endocrinol Metab. 97:2315-2324

28. Teiten M-H, et al, 2010. Chemopreventive potential of curcumin in prostate cancer. Genes Nutrition 5:61-74

In the next section we cover your output strategies of exercise and training to undermine prostate cancer progression. Training will help fully utilise the benefits from your improved input choices as you build a cancer-hostile prostate gland. Remember that each strategy reinforces the others in the quest to sabotage your cancer.

OUTPUT

Activity, Exercise and Training

All of us are active. We get out of bed and do things such as showering, cooking, gardening, shopping and working. Activities are good for us. They are much better than not being active but activities are not exercise.

Exercise occurs when your body systems respond to increased demand and lift their workload. Walking is an activity until you increase the speed or incline to demand more internal effort and cross the exercise threshold. You will feel the changes such as higher heart rate, deeper and faster breathing, perhaps some perspiration and flushing to disperse heat from working muscles and then fatigue as your energy stores become depleted.

These physiological changes are short lived, your body returning to its resting state on all measures soon after the exercise is completed. This return to idling is called homeostasis and reflects the body's preference for a minimal energy spend for any given level of activity or inactivity. Which is why 'activity' is not 'exercise' until you up the intensity.

Training is another level beyond exercise. Training is the result of repeated bouts of exercise that prompt long term changes (adaptations) within our body to enable us to perform more efficiently at a higher level. Exercise adaptations are temporary changes in physiological performance. Training adaptations are long term changes in body structure and function that prepare us for higher levels of performance.

Training harnesses the benefits of frequent exercising and transforms them into stronger muscles, more elastic blood vessels, a more competent heart, more efficient lungs, more resilient sinews and denser bone structure. Exercise can't do this unless it is repeated frequently enough to provoke the body to make internal changes to structure and function to improve performance long term. In maths -

Activity x Intensity = Exercise
Exercise x Frequency = Training

Understanding this is important when using physical activity as a tool for managing prostate cancer. You will need to be a frequent exerciser to power your training program.

This section outlines what training is required for exercise to help manage prostate cancer. The benefits will flow beyond your prostate by reducing your health risks from other cancers, cardiovascular disease, diabetes, osteoporosis, sarcopenia (muscle loss), dementia and other causes of cognitive decline. Prostate cancer may be the trigger to get healthy, fit and clear about what is important in your life.

> 'There is overwhelming evidence that appropriate exercise is safe and well tolerated in cancer survivors' [7]

Not only is exercise safe for cancer survivors, it helps undermine your prostate cancer, strengthens your immune system, maintains muscle and bone and gets you out of the house. We will look at a range of exercise and activities and it will be up to you to convert them into training.

Despite the evidence, health professionals are commonly unable or unwilling to introduce physical activity as a cancer managing strategy for patients. Research suggests this is partly due to lack of knowledge[1] but also assumptions they make about cancer survivors' energy reserves and interest or past history with physical activity.[2] Another reason given by health professionals was an inability to provide exercise programs due to lack of funding or other resources.[2]

Do not wait until physical activity is suggested by your medical team, instead take the lead and ask them when can you start, seek out appropriate and safe programs that interest you, tell them you are keen and ask them for medical clearance to begin. Then turn up.

Walking

This is the simplest training program of all - minimal equipment required and you can do it anywhere at most times of the day. You can add walking as an exercise to your life or you can integrate it into activities you already do.

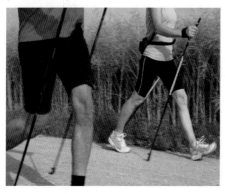

Ensure you have appropriate footwear - well constructed and supportive, cushioned and comfortable, weather-proof and stable as needed. Then open the door and start walking. If it is a new activity, build it gradually by walking 10 minutes out, turn around and walk back - 20 minutes done. After a week of daily walks, you can stretch it by doing an extra five minutes outwards and back. Another week and you increase to 30 minutes out for a total of one hour each session.

To make it an exercise, push the intensity a little by increasing the speed of walking, add a hill or two or wear a backpack with a couple of books or water bottles on board. You will know when it becomes an exercise by your increased breathing rate and depth, perspiration and higher heart rate. The recommended level is an intensity you would score as between 6 and 8 on a 10 point exertion scale, where 10 points is very exhausting and zero is thinking about putting your walking shoes on. Six to eight exertion points puts you in the heavy to very heavy exertion range. Slightly beyond your comfort zone is another way of rating it.

Walking intensity is important. A study on prostate tumour angiogenesis showed a higher walking speed was associated with a 48% decreased risk of prostate cancer recurrence compared with walking at an 'easy pace'.[3]

Additionally, a pre-diagnosis walking speed of greater than 4.8kph (3mph) is a predictor of reduced risk of developing lethal prostate cancer.[4] Maintaining a brisk walking pace may inhibit prostate cancer progression.

To convert your efforts into training, ensure you walk at least four days out of every seven. Five is better.

For many men, walking just for walking is pointless, boring and hard to sustain for weeks or months. So how can you make it more interesting? This will depend on your personal interests and motivations but here are some suggestions:

- Listen to an audio track with earbuds. Choose upbeat music that invites you to keep up, or a podcast of interest.
- Walk regularly with a friend you don't want to let down and who won't fail you either. They need to walk at your exercise pace, it won't help if you have to reduce intensity for them.
- Vary your walks, drive to a different start/finish point. Build a library of different walks and rotate them or throw a dice to decide on tomorrow's walk.
- Give your walk a purpose. Walk to a store to purchase the morning paper or a coffee shop where you can pause for refreshment before making the return journey. Walk to a friend's house or your doctor's office (always impressive).
- Use a tracker app or pedometer to log your distances walked, then add the daily distances together to get a total and apply this total to a target distance. The target might be walking across your home state or country, or from Chicago to Los Angeles on Route 66 or some other epic journey that stimulates your imagination.

A study of prostate cancer patients showed that walking for a total of 7 or more hours per week had a better cancer outcome than those men who walked less than 30 minutes per week.[5] There is a huge gap between these two levels where the benefits are not measurable. Which is no reason not to start and then build up to 7 hours per week.

If long walks are unappealing or don't fit your work/family schedules, you can complete the same total training time in smaller bursts. To your cardiovascular system, a daily one hour exercise walk is no different health-wise from four fifteen-minute exercise walks through the day, or six ten-minute walks. Look for opportunities to walk briskly during your normal day even for short bursts.

- Take the stairs for one floor then get the elevator. Next week, two floors then the elevator.
- Dodge the crowd by not using the escalator or moving walkway at airports, railway stations or shopping malls.
- Walk when you are on the phone at home or office.
- Convert a static meeting into a walking meeting: 'Walk with me'.

Cardiovascular or Aerobic Training

Walking is not the only option for training your cardiovascular system and improving heart efficiency, blood vessel elasticity, blood pressure, lung function and energy metabolism (release, utilisation and removal of waste products). Other options include jogging, running, swimming, aerobic classes in a gym or pool, paddling or rowing, cycling (stationary or mobile), boxing to music or any other activity that gets your heart rate up and holds it for 20 minutes or so. Nice thought, but sex generally won't make the cut and it's not the time for watching the clock.

Which activity you choose will be a function of many factors:

Cost - start up costs for equipment, joining fee, footwear and apparel. Ongoing costs for membership fees, travel and parking.

Availability - all you need for walking is a door to leave the building, other options may need a pool (heated, undercover), river or beach, cycle trails or access at times you are free.

Experience - what you have done previously may be safer and more skilled. Do you already have the equipment you need (kayak, cycle, swim goggles)?

Enjoyment - you have to enjoy the exercise or you won't turn it into training. You won't enjoy every session but over time you should enjoy the results and the improved fitness and health. Mixing your exercise modes can prolong enthusiasm and avoid boring repetition. For example, cycle two days per week, walk briskly two other days and swim on one day.

Resistance Training

This is different from 'resistance to training'. Using loads like free weights or equipment resistance machines to increase the resistance to movement is called resistance training (or doing weights).

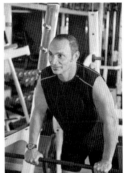

These exercises stress the muscles, sinews (tendons and fascia) and bones as you lift, push, pull, curl, dip, extend or hold against the load. With repeated episodes of controlled stress (load), muscles will build strength, tendons will become more resilient and bones will thicken as they lay down calcium. These changes happen in weeks, months and years respectively.

The preservation or regaining of muscle strength for men with prostate cancer is an important element in their quality of life.[6]

Which usually means we need to do targeted resistance training because our occupational or recreational activities do not qualify as strength training in terms of intensity or frequency. Perhaps, when younger, you worked physically hard every day but were promoted to a more supervisory role or changed jobs into a less active position. Or maybe you have retired by choice or medical necessity and mis-interpreted this transition as a reason to stop being active.

The guidelines for maximising the contribution of resistance training to sabotage prostate cancer progression have been established by Australian researchers.[7] The threshold numbers are -

> The minimum effective dose for resistance training in prostate cancer survivors is:
> - two or more sessions per week,
> - involving three or more sets of 6-8 exercises
> - at an intensity of 6-10 repeated maximums (RM).

Unless you have a history of structured resistance training this may require some decoding.

Sessions per week is the number of times you perform your resistance training program.

Sets refers to the number of times you complete 6-10 movement repetitions of each exercise.

Repetitions is the number of movements you perform in each set.

Repeated Maximum (RM) is the intensity measure where the number of repetitions is the maximum number you can perform before fatigue prevents you from continuing. One RM means the load can only be lifted once before you are too fatigued to perform a second repetition. Six RM means the load is sufficiently heavy to restrict you to six repetitions before fatigue prevents the seventh. Ten RM will involve a lighter load that allows you to complete 10 repetitions before fatigue.

Notice that the intensity resistance training is based on your fatigue rate which is determined by the resistance load. This is irrespective of the nature of the resistance - it could be a free weight (dumbbell, barbell or kettlebell), machine generated hydraulic resistance, elastic resistance using bands or water resistance in a pool.

If you are able to complete more than 10 repetitions against the load you are not in an optimal dose zone for a strength training response. You should increase the load (resistance) until you are in the 6-10 RM fatigue zone. ***Provided the heavier load is safe for you.***

Prostate cancer tends to be a disease of older men so the probability of you having physical or medical limitations when starting a strength program after your diagnosis is higher. You may be carrying old sporting or work injuries, arthritic joints, tendon wear and tear or medical conditions (heart or respiratory disease, diabetes) that limit your workload. It is safer to start with light resistance and gradually build as your tolerance improves. Continuity is more important than courage.

> It is important you are cleared by your physician or medical team before commencing a resistance training program.
>
> It is also recommended that your program is supervised by a fitness or exercise professional to ensure you learn correct technique and your safe starting loads can be assessed.

When you start a resistance training program, it is normal to begin with lighter loads which may feel easy and don't fatigue you within the target zone. Don't be concerned as the initial emphasis is on safe and efficient exercise technique, your movement skills and tolerance to loading. Once you have demonstrated your skills and common sense and shown early improvement, the loading can be gradually increased moving into the strength training zone of 6-10 repetitions in each set.

The type of resistance exercise you choose is less important for sabotaging prostate cancer than how disciplined you are in turning up regularly and pushing yourself into the training zone.

Examples of resistance training

Body Weight Exercises	Free Weight Exercises	Machine Exercises
Press Ups	Lateral Shoulder Raises	Lat Pull Downs
Triceps Dips	Biceps Curls	Leg Press
Chin Ups	Overhead Press	Pec Deck
Squats	Bench Press	Cable Rows

Circuit Training

This type of workout is a sequence of exercise stations each to be completed for a set time. The stations can include exercises for strength, agility, power, endurance, movement skills and balance. For more than 20 years I have used circuit training for older men to outwit the age-related changes associated with not training. The men in my groups have a range of medical conditions including prostate cancer, diabetes, arthritis, chronic back pain, hip and knee replacements, coronary artery disease, depression/anxiety, Parkinson's disease, stroke, sleep apnoea, dementia, lung disease, melanoma and dodgy shoulder tendons. Many of them have more than one from that list. All of them are on drugs. Not performance enhancing drugs (although they do help) but prescription medication for underlying health issues. Regular testing of these men shows retention of muscle mass, bone mass, strength, functional strength and agility. All of which would otherwise decline with age and/or inactivity.

In one circuit I use 26 exercise stations sequenced to provide strength work interspersed with aerobic bursts, spending one minute per station followed by a 15 second change over. This means a total of 26 minutes of working out with just over 6 minutes of change-over time on a 4:1 work/rest ratio. They are in and out of the gym in a little over 30 minutes, three times per week - efficient, varied and thorough.

When done well, participants get a cardiovascular training session peppered with strength training stations. It also means I can train up to 26 men at the same time. The quality of supervision to ensure safety for all participants plus effective training is paramount in a busy circuit session. If you ever feel you are not being sufficiently supervised let the staff know you would like more attention as you learn.

Flexibility

In my experience, many men find stretching and flexibility training a bit like walking - 'Sounds good, but why?' When you were an elite athlete (or at least had the potential) stretching had a purpose. If you still play sport or golf, you may find stretching remains useful for your performance, recovery or comfort.

However, if you haven't done much flexibility work in recent years a compelling reason to start arrived on the day you decided to adopt AS as your treatment plan. Stretching on its own won't sabotage prostate cancer directly but it will enable your body to better cope with the other physical activity demands you are about to start in your Output strategy.

As you begin your brisk walking program and your two or three days per week in the strength gym or circuit, you may find doing stretching exercises improves your ability to bend, lift, get off the floor, reach upwards, tie your shoe laces, get out of the car when arriving home and step into your pants without catching your toes eight times out of ten.

Your physical therapist, exercise or fitness professional can help with a simple, general purpose stretching program modified to suit your age and any warrior injuries from your youth. There are also many online resources but you will miss the supervision as you learn to do the stretch exercises correctly and safely.

When trying to gain flexibility, you should stretch every couple of days at least. Once you have achieved your goal you need only stretch thoroughly every five to seven days to maintain your range of mobility.

When stretching, it is usually more effective to apply the muscle stretch during your out-breath, easing into the stretch range as you slowly breathe out. Then hold the stretch for between 30 and 45 seconds while breathing normally and letting any tension ease away. Repeat each stretch at least twice in your session.

Yoga / Tai Chi / Pilates

There are many other exercise options and you may find them enjoyable, affordable and convenient but I hope you don't find them comfortable. If an exercise is comfortable it may only be an activity and certainly won't result in training.

Yoga, Tai Chi and Pilates are examples of exercise programs each having specific training potentials. Yoga is good for postural endurance, flexibility, breathing and muscle control. Tai Chi is excellent for balance, postural control, falls prevention and movement skills, Pilates is a training program for muscle recruitment, safe movement patterns and postural endurance. Each has benefits but typically none is a cardiovascular or resistance training program of sufficient intensity to be the entirety of your output during your prostate cancer sabotage project. Yoga and Tai Chi add an element of mindfulness training to the

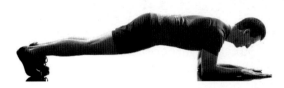

The Plank - a body weight core strength-endurance exercise common to many programs

routine as you focus internally and filter the external noise of life. This doubling down may be useful if you are struggling to find time or energy to participate.

These programs can add variety and other physiological benefits to complement your training program and may help with recovery after intense physical sessions. They may also be quite sociable and add to your quality of life. Try them to discover if they are a good fit for you.

My colleague, Jo Milios, has developed 'JOGA 4 Men' which raises funds for a prostate cancer foundation. Her program is available on CD or USB at www.prost.com.au.

Ejaculation

Come again? Evidence suggests increased frequency of ejaculation might provide some protection against prostate cancer. Researchers have proposed a figure of 21 times per month as the exercise dose, but are not sure how it helps.[8] Suggestions include regular emptying of the seminal vesicles and prostate might reduce toxins (a 'use-by' theory) or perhaps the muscle activity promotes blood flow into the gland. Maybe healthier men (better diet and physical activity) have more sexual activity and less prostate cancer but one doesn't cause the other.

This doesn't mean having intercourse 21 times per month. Ejaculation does not require an assistant but if help is offered you can accept on tenuous medical grounds. If you went to the gym 21 times per month it would be considered training, so this is a high performance training activity with benefits. No, don't do it at the gym. Frequent ejaculation does not increase your risk of prostate cancer, so that's good news.

OUTPUT SUMMARY

Do No Harm

- Seek medical clearance from your GP or physician before undertaking a new training regime.
- Seek professional supervision of any resistance training or high intensity program to ensure safe technique and sensible progressions.

Be Realistic

If you have not trained for some time, just get used to turning up regularly and doing something. You can increase the intensity later. Don't go too hard too early.

Once in the routine, make sure you have elements of strength, cardio-vascular, flexibility in the mix and at a frequency and intensity to create changes in your body and mind.

Enjoy It

After an intitial transition period, your training program should be something you look forward to. If not, you need to mix it up a bit, to make it more varied, sociable or challenging.

Don't Stop

Training effects only remain as long as you are exercising them. Reducing or stopping the program will lead to de-training, which is the opposite of training. Also known as disappointing.

Output References

1. Cantwell M et al, 2018. Healthcare professionals' knowledge and practice of physical activity promotion in cancer care. Challenges and solutions. European J of Cancer Care 278e:12795

2. Haussmann A et al, 2018. What hinders health professionals in promoting physical activity towards cancer patients? The influencing role of healthcare professionals' concerns, perceived patient characteristics and perceived structural factors. European J of Cancer Care 27:e12853

3. Sanchis-Gomar F et al, 2015 Physical inactivity and low fitness deserve more attention to alter cancer risk and prognosis. Cancer Prev Res. 8:105-110.

4. Van Blarigan E, 2015. Physical activity and prostate tumor vessel morphology: data from the health professionals follow-up study. Cancer Prev Research 8(10):962-7

5. Friedenrich C et al 2016. Physical activity and cancer outcomes - a precision medicine approach. J. Clinical Cancer Research 22(19):4716

6. Morishita S et al 2018. Cancer survivors exhibit a different relationship between muscle strength and health-related quality of life/fatigue compared to healthy subjects. European J of Cancer Care 27:e12856

7. Newton R & Galvao D, 2013. Exercise medicine for prostate cancer. Eur Rev Aging Physical Activity. 10:41-45.

8. Rider J. et al 2015. Ejaculation frequency and risk of prostate cancer: updated results from the health professionals follow-up study. J of Urology 193(4S):e148.

We have completed the three Playbook strategies to keep your prostate gland: throughput, input and output.

The next chapter highlights the most common way it all goes belly up for men: premature congratulations.

PREMATURE CONGRATULATIONS

One of the most dangerous aspects of starting a new program, when you are strongly motivated by fear and enthusiasm, is early success. Especially if that early success has come with only a moderate effort as is often the case when there is plenty of room for improvement due to your starting point.

This early success gets you thinking that you are going too hard, too early. Perhaps you see an opportunity to take your foot off the accelerator.

Case Hypothetical #1

Let's say you want to lose 10kg in weight. You make some changes to your eating plan, perhaps counting kilojoules, intermittent fasting, giving up alcohol or dairy products. Over the first week you lose one kilogram, in the second week you lose an additional 1.5kg. Now you are 25% toward your ultimate goal and finding it pretty easy. Brilliant, a few simple changes and the weight starts falling away.

This early success prompts a rethink of your strategy and you start backsliding into an occasional glass of red or putting milk in your coffee again. Secure in your new found capacity to get results any old time, why should you deprive yourself to such an extent? In fact, you deserve a treat for doing so well. Welcome to 'Premature Congratulations'.

Over the third week you gain 1kg. but don't panic: weight loss is never linear (you tell yourself). By the end of week four you are back at your starting weight and wondering if the whole process is really worth it. After all you lost weight and then it came back, conveniently overlooking your role in the 'failure' of the program.

When it comes to weight loss you can't really celebrate until your have remained at or below your target for at least three months.

Case Hypothetical #2

You commit to increasing your physical exercise level by walking every morning, cycling or swimming a couple of times per week or taking out a gym membership.

You start your new exercise program full of enthusiasm and commitment to make it a training program. Only to discover the new program is difficult to fit into your work-life timetable. You have to get up earlier, arrive home from work later, see less of your family and sacrifice social opportunities just to get it done.

Your training program, which you know you need, is proving quite a struggle, not only to fit into your timetable but it is also unpleasant (it hurts, you sweat and get tired) and it demands feeding in the form of new shoes, clothing, equipment and recurring effort.

Nevertheless, you battle on making the adjustments necessary to fit this into your life, work, home and resources. And you start to feel healthier and have more energy and sleep better. You become more productive at work and more popular at home, despite (or because?) you are there less frequently. Well done you. And really, how hard was it? Once you started it just all came together. So perhaps you can ease off a bit and only walk every second day, or drop the gym to twice per week instead of four sessions.

You are again suffering from a 'Premature Congratulation'.

This phenomenon is very common and I speak from personal experience where early success gives a misguided sense of control over the hoped-for outcome and I take my foot off the change accelerator only to see the early results evaporate.

What is the treatment?

We are both the problem and the solution. We need to overcome the human tendency to equate prior success with an assurance of future outcomes. It doesn't work in financial investment and it certainly doesn't work in modifying long term behavioural habits.

Acknowledging you are experiencing premature congratulation is the first step in overcoming it. But just knowing about it is not enough.

You need to anticipate its arrival. You may believe premature congratulation only happens to other men; but they are all thinking the same, which means many of us will be totally wrong. We all need strategies to prevent any backsliding, here are some suggestions.

Keep Score - keep a record of every time you stick to the new plan. If you are on a new eating program, give yourself a tick for every day you get it right, and mark yourself hard if you lapse on a particular day. Keep recording the results for three months especially if you are struggling. It is really important to remind yourself every day whether you are doing your part in the program. Everyday without a tick is an opportunity to do better tomorrow. A prompt to regroup, buckle-down, focus, sacrifice, go hungry, miss things and get a tick tomorrow.

If you are on an activity program, score yourself a win for every session you complete. Be honest and only score a win for those sessions where you not only turned up but did the work at the intensity and duration required. Turning up is important but doing the work earns the win.

Buddy Up - Why should you suffer alone? Find a companion (friend, family, workmate) who would also benefit from the output intervention and work together to get double results. He or she doesn't need to have prostate cancer, their motivation can be different. You can jointly research the program, set up a recording sheet, organise a meeting time and place on a regular basis, share the transport, keep an eye on each other and wear matching outfits (too far?).

The idea is to hold each other accountable, not through a formal performance review, but through an expectation that you are in this together and knowing that a mate is expecting you to turn up can often make the difference from being a no-show when everything is not perfect.

Compete - sort of. The problem with the traditional concept of competing is that someone wins and someone loses. Which is great if you are the winner but really sucks if you are not. What we need is a way of competing where everyone comes out a winner and I don't just mean they get a medal for turning up, they all actually win in some way.

If you are on a girth reduction program (probably reducing your food input) you buddy up with a mate and compete to see who can lose 10cm and keep it off for two months. If your mate gets there first (in six weeks, say) that's great - congratulate him and ask how he did it. Then keep going. The target hasn't changed and you haven't failed if you are slimmer than when you began the challenge. You are just not finished yet. Don'stop now, that would be premature congratulations.

Another way to compete in a collaborative way is to reward both of you for shared achievement. If the initial target was 10cm or 10 kg each, you could instead work together to achieve a combined loss of 20cm or 20kg. One of you might do the lion's share (and perhaps he needed to) but you both get to celebrate the final goal and feel like winners together.

WEIGHT LOSS

I haven't discussed losing weight as a strategy for prostate cancer sabotage because it isn't. Weight loss is an outcome from a successful modification of throughput, input and output: it is the feedback from your body that what you are doing is working. Not all men with prostate cancer need to lose weight and some may gain as their muscle mass improves. Establishing healthy habits enables your body to move toward its preferred state.

This Playbook is not a weight loss program, it is a strategic guide to suppressing the development and growth of prostate cancer. Any weight optimisation or slimming of girth is a bonus outcome.

Following the advice in this Playbook will help you move toward your ideal weight range and stay there. The benefits will include:

- reduced inflammatory load
- better hunger regulation
- easier physical training
- improved sleep
- better self-esteem
- mastery over your health decisions
- and for your prostate gland: **Keep It. Healthy.**

GLOSSARY

Active Surveillance (AS)
An undetermined period between diagnosis of prostate cancer and beginning curative treatment during which the specialists monitor for changes in the character of the cancer and the patient actively strives to inhibit and sabotage the cancer in the hope of avoiding surgery or other invasive treatments.

ADT
Androgen Deprivation Therapy (ADT) is a pharmacological treatment to decrease the level and effects of male hormones (androgens) generated in a man's body. Previously female hormones (oestrogens) were used but this is largely discontinued due to the side effects. Current drugs work either on the pituitary gland to reduce the hormone message to produce androgens or at the take up point where they block the action of the androgen at receptor sites.

Angiogenesis
The budding and extension of arterial blood vessels into a mass of cells. In this case into a prostate cancer site. Nutrition, oxygen and clearance of waste through these vessels allows the cancer to grow.

Anti-oxidant
A chemical or molecule that buffers free radicals and restores chemical balance. It may be produced internally or acquired through diet or supplementation.

Brachytherapy
Precision insertion of tiny radioactive beads directly into the prostate gland where they deliver a low intensity but sustained irradiation to inhibit and kill cancer cells. These remain in situ permanently with minimal side effects. Only suitable for localised, lower intensity cancer.

CyberKnife ®
Another form of radiotherapy using robotic radiosurgery treatment for cancer where radiation is indicated. A new delivery of radiation in which the convergent radiation beams alter alignment to reduce collateral damage to adjacent healthy tissue or if the target zone moves. Sounds like surgery but isn't.

Doubling Time
The time it takes for a PSA score to double. Many men experience a benign enlargement of their prostate as they age and the bigger prostate leaks more PSA into the bloodstream. A doubling time of less than five years is considered abnormal and requires investigation. Abbreviated to PSAD.

DRE
Digital Rectal Examination (DRE) is exactly that: a gloved digit (finger) is used in the rectum to feel for any abnormalities on the rear wall of the prostate gland. Should be performed by qualified practitioners only.

Epigenetics
The science of gene-switches whereby a genetic instruction remains inactive until the appropriate epigenetic switch is activated. Until then the expression of the gene is a potential effect. Activating the switch increases the chance of the instruction being followed.

Gleason Score
Based on analysis of biopsy samples taken from the prostate, two numbers are reported. The first is the Gleason grade (1 to 5) for the most predominant pattern of cancer cells in a sample, and the second is the grade for the second most predominant pattern. These two are added together for a Gleason Score which expresses the likely chance of the cancer growing and spreading beyond the prostate gland. The score is used to help determine the most appropriate treatment. If cancer is detected on the biopsy the lowest score possible is 6 (low grade). Score of 8 and over indicate a fast-growing cancer. Interpreting a score of 7 varies depending if it is a 3+4 (more favorable) or a 4+3 (less favourable). The Gleason is used in conjunction with other test results.

Grade Group System
This is replacing the Gleason system as a more reliable grading of aggressiveness of the cancer. Grades are Goup 1 (slow-growing and less agressive), Group 2-3 (faster growing and moderately aggressive) and Group 4-5 (fast growing and aggressive). This still uses the Gleason number from a biopsy to group the cancer.

MRI
Magnetic Resonance Imaging (MRI) is a radiological imaging system particularly suited to assessing soft tissues such as a prostate gland. Manipulation of the magnetic waves and of the resultant images can improve accuracy of diagnostic interpretation. The machine is large, noisy and claustrophobic for some.

Oxidative Stress
The build up in the body of oxidative ions (free radicals) disturbing the chemical environment in which your body performs the millions of reactions every second. Occurs when your defense system is unable to neutralise your normal oxidation by-product or when increased production overwhelms your capacity to neutralise (buffer). End result is a decrease in immune system effectiveness.

PHI
Prostate Health Index (PHI) is a calculation using all three forms of PSA (total, free and p2) that are found in blood tests arriving at a single score that expresses the likely progression of the cancer during active surveillance. It is another useful tool when assessing risk and need for biopsy or treatment.

PI-RADS

Prostate Imaging Reporting and Data System (PI-RADS) is a structure reporting scheme for evaluating prostate cancer used prior to treatment. The score between 1 (low chance of clinically significant cancer) and 5 (very high chance) is calculated based on multiparametric MRI images.

PSA

Prostate Specific Antigen (PSA) is a normal product of prostate activity added to the semen. Its role is to release the sperm cells from the seminal fluid. PSA also leaks into th e bloodstream where it can be detected on testing and used to demonstrate prostate gland activity levels and irritability. Elevated PSA is not diagnostic of cancer.

Radical Prostatectomy

Surgical removal of the prostate gland, its capsule, embedded nerves and blood vessels, prostatic urethra and possibly its muscular sphincters. Can be an open, laparascopic (keyhole) or robot-assisted procedure. Side effects can include incontinence, erectile dysfunction and depression. Full eradication of the cancer is not guaranteed.

Radiation therapy - External Beam

Externally applied beams of radiation targetted to intersect (cross) at the site of the cancer. This delivers a fatal dose of radiation to those cells and any others close enough to share the high intensity. Usually a course of many daily treatments. Side effects include adjacent tissue necrosis (death), fatigue and depression.

TNM System

This is a method to express the stage of the cancer, which indicates how likely it is to spread within and beyond the prostate gland. Numbers are assigned for the size of the tumour (T), whether the cancer has spread to nearby lymph nodes (N) and whether the cancer has spread to bones or other organs (M). The scores are combined to arrive at a Stage 1-2 (contained and early), Stage 3 (larger and spread to nearby organs) or Stage 4 (spread to distant parts or bones.metastasized).

SpaceOAR ®

A gel that is injected into the space between the prostate and the rectum prior to commencing radiation therapy. This provides protection against over-radiating the rectum and causing burns or scarring. The water based gel remains in place during the course of radiotherapy and is slowly absorbed by the body over time.

Training - effect

The changes your body components make in response to an appropriate load of physical activity. Training effects include increased muscle and bone mass, strength, flexibility, agility , balance, skill patterns, and continence.

Watchful Waiting

An undetermined period following diagnosis during which a man continues to indulge lifestyle behaviours that resulted in him developing prostate cancer in the first place. Only to be amazed when it gets worse and demands treatment.

SURVEILLANCE RECORD

Date	Procedure	PSA	Gleason

This table is to enter your test results if you are on Active Surveillance or if you are still in screening mode. This 'at a glance' tracking of key numbers and actions may prove useful when determining your next steps.

Other	Questions	Action Required

INDEX

WHY NOT USE CRAIG ALLINGHAM AS GUEST SPEAKER FOR YOUR NEXT CONFERENCE OR EVENT?

Craig Allingham is renowned as an expert in men's physical health and performance.

His training in physiotherapy, sports science and men's health collide with his Executive MBA to make him an ideal speaker to link health, performance and results with a liberal sprinkling of humour. Ask him about the 'Give a Shit Index' for men.

Craig has keynoted international conferences in Australia, New Zealand. the UK, Netherlands and USA. He is an experienced and trained speaker with an ability to adapt content to match the interests of the audience and the goals of the organisers.

His experience at four Olympic Games in high performance medicine provides stories and laughs to underpin his more serious messages of how health impacts on success.

Contact Craig through
info@redsok.com
His web presence is at
www.craigallingham.com

ALSO BY CRAIG

The Prostate Recovery MAP

Men's Action Plan 2

For men who have undergone treatment for prostate cancer and want to regain their continence and erectile function.

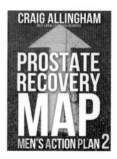

Based on Craig's years of clinical experience in men's health physiotherapy and sports rehabilitation. He guides you through the stages of activating, strengthening and training your pelvic floor including an optional Master Class for the pelvic floor athlete.

Thousands of men have benefited from this practical and logical program.

Get yours at

www.prostaterecoverymap.com

or bookstores in Australia and NZ